CHAIR YOGA FOR SENIORS OVER 60

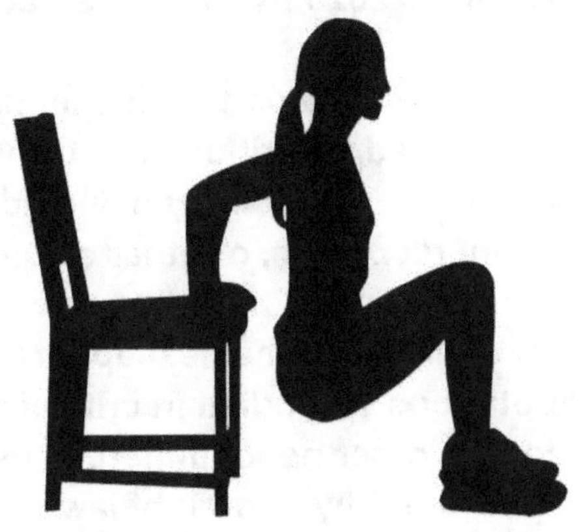

Embracing Balance, Flexibility, and Serenity in Every Pose

By
Charlotte Scott

TABLE OF CONTENTS

INTRODUCTION..5

Chapter 1..7

Definition and origins of chair yoga...................7

Benefits of chair yoga for seniors..............10

Addressing common concerns and misconceptions............................13

Chapter 2...17

Understanding Seniors' Health Needs............17

Common health issues faced by seniors.. 17

How chair yoga can address health concerns...21

Importance of flexibility, balance, and mental well-being in seniors.....................25

Chapter 3..29

Getting Started with Chair Yoga.....................29

Choosing tho right chair and space for practicing...29

Warm-up exercises tailored for seniors.....32

Breathing techniques for relaxation and focus..35

Chapter 4..42

Chair Yoga Poses for Mobility and Flexibility.. 42

Seated yoga poses to improve joint

flexibility...........................42

Gentle stretches to increase mobility........ 46

Modifications for different fitness levels.... 51

Chapter 5.. **57**

Chair Yoga for Balance and Stability...............57

Balancing poses to enhance stability........ 57

Techniques to improve posture and core strength.. 62

Fall prevention exercises........................... 69

Chapter 6.. **76**

Chair Yoga for Pain Relief............................. 76

Yoga poses to alleviate common pains..... 76

Breathing and meditation techniques for pain management..................................... 81

Partner stretches and massages for pain relief.. 87

Chapter 7.. **92**

Chair Yoga for Mental and Emotional Well-being... 92

Mindfulness and meditation exercises...... 92

Promoting mental clarity and emotional resilience... 102

Chapter 8.. **108**

Chair Yoga for Specific Health Conditions.... 108

Chair yoga tailored for specific health issues 108

Poses and practices to complement medical treatments.. 114

Precautions and contraindications for various conditions....................................118

Chapter 9.. **125**

Chair Yoga for Daily Living..............................125

Incorporating chair yoga into daily routines... 125

Chair yoga for better sleep.....................131

Yoga practices for energy and vitality......136

Chapter 10... **143**

Building a Supportive Chair Yoga Community.... 143

Creating chair yoga groups and classes for seniors...143

Encouraging social interaction and support.. 149

Conclusion.. **156**

Recap of key lessons and practices............ 156

Encouragement for ongoing chair yoga practice...161

INTRODUCTION

In the hushed pages of this book, we embark on a transformative odyssey, where the creak of bones and the whisper of breath meet the power of mindfulness and movement. Within these chapters, you will find more than just a guide; you will discover a sanctuary tailored for the golden souls seeking vitality, serenity, and an enduring connection with their bodies.

Imagine a world where every stretch is a dance, every breath is a melody, and every moment is a celebration of the strength within. This book, woven with care and expertise, unlocks the secrets of Chair Yoga, offering a pathway to enhanced flexibility, improved balance, and a renewed sense of inner peace. Beyond the physical postures, it becomes a journey of self-discovery, a conduit to a deeper understanding of the body-mind connection that transcends the boundaries of age.

But this book is more than just a manual; it is a beacon of hope, an assurance that life, even in its later stages, can be vibrant, fulfilling, and joyous. Through the meticulously crafted poses, breathing exercises, and meditative practices, you will find a renewed sense of purpose, a resurgence of energy, and a profound shift in perspective.

So, dear reader, if you find yourself at the crossroads of time, where the years have painted the canvas of your life with a myriad of hues, allow this book to be your guiding light. Embrace the wisdom of Chair Yoga, and let it infuse your days with vitality, your nights with peace, and your heart with boundless joy. Your journey to a healthier, happier, and more harmonious life begins here. Welcome to a world where age is not a limitation but a canvas for a beautiful, enduring masterpiece.

Chapter 1

Definition and origins of chair yoga

Chair yoga, a gentle form of yoga practiced while sitting on a chair or using a chair for support, has gained popularity worldwide, especially among seniors and individuals with limited mobility. This innovative practice adapts traditional yoga postures into seated or modified versions, making it accessible to a broader range of people.

Origins:

The origins of chair yoga can be traced back to the ancient discipline of yoga, which originated in India over 5,000 years ago. Traditional yoga encompasses a wide array of physical, mental, and spiritual practices, aiming to promote overall well-being and self-realization. Over the centuries, yoga evolved, and in the modern context, various yoga styles and adaptations emerged to cater to different needs.

The concept of chair yoga as we know it today began to take shape in the late 20th century. Yoga teachers and healthcare professionals started exploring ways to make yoga accessible to seniors and individuals with physical limitations. They recognized the need for a practice that could provide the benefits of yoga, such as improved flexibility, balance, and relaxation, without the need to get down on the floor. As a result, chair yoga was developed, offering a safe and effective way for people of all ages and abilities to experience the positive effects of yoga.

Definition:

Chair yoga is a gentle form of yoga that modifies traditional yoga poses to be practiced while sitting on a chair or using a chair for support. It combines gentle stretching, deep breathing, and relaxation techniques to enhance flexibility, balance, and mental focus. Unlike other forms of yoga, chair yoga eliminates the need for complex transitions or getting up and down from the floor, making it suitable for seniors, individuals with disabilities, and anyone seeking a gentle yet effective exercise routine.

Key Features of Chair Yoga:

- **Seated Poses:** Chair yoga focuses on a variety of seated poses, allowing practitioners to work on different muscle groups and joints while remaining comfortably seated. These poses are designed to improve flexibility and range of motion.
- **Breath Awareness:** One of the fundamental aspects of chair yoga is breath awareness.

Practitioners are guided to synchronize their movements with their breath, promoting relaxation and enhancing the mind-body connection.

- **Use of Props:** Chairs are used as props to support and enhance yoga poses. Practitioners can hold onto the chair back for balance, use it for seated forward bends, or incorporate it into standing poses for additional stability.
- **Adaptability:** Chair yoga is highly adaptable, making it suitable for individuals with various physical conditions, including arthritis, chronic pain, or mobility issues. Poses can be modified further to meet individual needs and limitations.

Benefits of Chair Yoga:

Chair yoga offers a myriad of benefits, including improved flexibility, enhanced balance and coordination, reduced stress and anxiety, increased joint mobility, and better posture. Regular practice can also contribute to pain management, improved circulation, and a sense of overall well-being.

In summary, chair yoga is a holistic and inclusive approach to yoga practice, embracing individuals of all ages and physical abilities. Its gentle yet effective techniques make it a valuable tool for promoting physical, mental, and emotional wellness, making yoga accessible to everyone, regardless of their limitations or age.

Benefits of chair yoga for seniors

Chair yoga offers a plethora of physical, mental, and emotional benefits specifically tailored to the needs of seniors. This gentle form of yoga, practiced with the aid of a chair, provides a safe and effective way for older adults to enhance their overall well-being. Here's a detailed look at the numerous advantages chair yoga offers to seniors:

1. Improved Flexibility:
Chair yoga incorporates gentle stretches and movements, enhancing seniors' flexibility without putting strain on their joints. Increased flexibility contributes to improved range of motion, making everyday activities easier and reducing the risk of injuries.

2. Enhanced Balance and Stability:
Seniors often face challenges related to balance and stability, which can lead to falls and injuries. Chair yoga focuses on balance-enhancing poses, helping seniors develop a stronger sense of stability and coordination. This can significantly reduce the risk of falls and improve overall mobility.

3. Pain Relief and Management:

Many seniors suffer from chronic pain conditions such as arthritis or lower back pain. Chair yoga's gentle movements and stretches can alleviate pain and discomfort. Regular practice helps in strengthening muscles, reducing stiffness, and promoting better posture, leading to effective pain management.

4. Stress Reduction:

Chair yoga incorporates deep breathing exercises and relaxation techniques, which are known to reduce stress and promote a sense of calm. Seniors often experience stress due to various factors like health concerns or lifestyle changes. Regular practice of chair yoga can help seniors manage stress levels and improve their overall quality of life.

5. Increased Circulation:

Chair yoga includes gentle movements of the limbs and deep breathing, promoting better blood circulation throughout the body. Improved circulation is essential for cardiovascular health, reducing the risk of heart-related issues and promoting overall vitality.

6. Enhanced Respiratory Function:

The focus on breathing techniques in chair yoga helps seniors expand their lung capacity and improve respiratory function. This is particularly beneficial for seniors with respiratory conditions like asthma or COPD. Proper breathing techniques can increase oxygen intake and promote better lung health.

7. Better Posture:

Chair yoga emphasizes body awareness and proper alignment. Seniors often struggle with poor posture, which can lead to back pain and discomfort. Through chair yoga, seniors learn to sit and stand with correct posture, reducing strain on the spine and promoting a healthier back.

8. Mental Clarity and Relaxation:

Chair yoga incorporates mindfulness and meditation practices, enhancing mental clarity and promoting relaxation. Seniors can experience reduced anxiety, improved focus, and a sense of inner peace through regular practice. These benefits contribute to better mental and emotional well-being.

9. Social Engagement:

Participating in chair yoga classes provides seniors with the opportunity to socialize and connect with others in a supportive environment. Feelings of loneliness and isolation are diminished by social contact, which is crucial for mental and emotional health.

10. Accessible Exercise:
One of the significant benefits of chair yoga is its accessibility. Seniors with limited mobility or physical disabilities can participate in chair yoga comfortably. The use of a chair provides stability, making the practice safe and inclusive for all seniors, regardless of their fitness level.

In summary, chair yoga offers a holistic approach to promoting the health and well-being of seniors. Its gentle yet effective techniques address the unique needs of older adults, providing them with a practical and enjoyable way to stay active, reduce stress, manage pain, and enhance their overall quality of life. Regular practice of chair yoga empowers seniors to age gracefully, maintaining their physical and mental vitality.

Addressing common concerns and misconceptions

As chair yoga gains popularity, it's essential to address common concerns and misconceptions that might deter individuals from trying this beneficial practice. By dispelling these myths, more people, including seniors and those with limited mobility, can confidently embrace chair yoga as a valuable part of their wellness routine.

1. "Yoga is Only for the Young and Flexible":
This misconception often prevents seniors from exploring yoga. Chair yoga, however, is specifically designed for individuals with diverse abilities. Its gentle approach makes it accessible to people of all ages, body types, and fitness levels, allowing seniors to enjoy the benefits of yoga without feeling intimidated.

2. "Chair Yoga Isn't a Real Workout":
While chair yoga may appear less intense than traditional yoga, it offers a comprehensive workout tailored to seniors' needs. It focuses on flexibility, balance, strength, and relaxation. The controlled movements and poses provide a gentle yet effective workout, improving muscle tone, joint mobility, and overall stamina.

3. "You Need Special Equipment":
The beauty of chair yoga lies in its simplicity. As the name suggests, all you need is a sturdy chair. No fancy equipment or attire is required. Participants can wear comfortable clothes and practice in any quiet space, making it convenient and accessible.

4. "It's Only for People with Limited Mobility":
While chair yoga is indeed accessible for those with limited mobility, it's not exclusive to them. Many able-bodied individuals, including office workers looking to relieve stress or individuals recovering from injuries, find chair yoga beneficial. The practice can be adapted to challenge participants at various fitness levels.

5. "Chair Yoga Isn't Relaxing":
Chair yoga incorporates relaxation techniques such as deep breathing, meditation, and mindfulness. These techniques encourage calmness, lessen tension, and improve mental clarity. Many participants find chair yoga to be deeply calming, providing both physical and mental relaxation.

6. "I'm Too Old for Yoga":
Yoga has no age limit, and chair yoga is especially well-suited for seniors. In fact, it can be highly beneficial for older adults, enhancing their flexibility, balance, and overall well-being. It's never too late to start practicing chair yoga, and many seniors find it empowering and rejuvenating.

7. "It's Just Sitting, How Can It Be Good for Me?
While chair yoga is practiced sitting on a chair, it involves dynamic movements and poses that engage

various muscle groups. It's not simply sitting; it's about mindful movement. The practice strengthens the core, improves posture, and enhances circulation, providing numerous physical benefits despite being seated.

8. "I Need to Be Spiritual or Religious to Practice Yoga":

Yoga is not tied to any specific religion or spirituality. While yoga has roots in ancient spiritual traditions, chair yoga classes typically focus on the physical aspects, breathing techniques, and relaxation. Participants are encouraged to focus on their own well-being, irrespective of their religious beliefs.

In conclusion, chair yoga is a versatile and inclusive practice suitable for everyone. By addressing these concerns and misconceptions, more individuals, especially seniors, can recognize the value of chair yoga in promoting physical health, mental well-being, and overall quality of life. It's a practice that celebrates the body's abilities and encourages a sense of empowerment, making it a valuable addition to anyone's fitness routine.

Chapter 2

Understanding Seniors' Health Needs

Common health issues faced by seniors

As individuals age, they often encounter a variety of health challenges. Seniors are more susceptible to certain medical conditions and illnesses due to the natural aging process and the wear and tear on the body over the years. Understanding these common health issues is crucial for both seniors and their caregivers, as it enables better management, prevention, and overall well-being in the elderly population. Here is a detailed overview of some of the most prevalent health concerns faced by seniors:

1. Cardiovascular Diseases:
Heart diseases such as coronary artery disease, heart failure, and hypertension become more common with age. Seniors are at a higher risk of heart attacks and strokes due to factors like high blood pressure,

high cholesterol, and reduced physical activity. Maintaining a heart-healthy diet, regular exercise, and managing stress are essential in preventing cardiovascular issues.

2. Arthritis:

Arthritis is a group of joint disorders causing inflammation, pain, stiffness, and decreased mobility. Osteoarthritis, the most common type, occurs when the cartilage that cushions the joints wears down over time. Rheumatoid arthritis, an autoimmune disorder, is another form. Exercise, weight management, and proper medical care help manage arthritis symptoms.

3. Osteoporosis:

Weakened bones that are more prone to fractures and breaks are the hallmark of osteoporosis. It's particularly prevalent in postmenopausal women. Adequate calcium and vitamin D intake, weight-bearing exercises, and certain medications can help prevent osteoporosis and reduce the risk of fractures.

4. Diabetes:

Type 2 diabetes, often related to lifestyle factors, becomes more common with age. Seniors with diabetes must manage their blood sugar levels through diet, exercise, medication, and regular monitoring to prevent complications such as nerve damage, vision problems, and heart disease.

5. Dementia and Alzheimer's Disease:
Dementia, including Alzheimer's disease, affects memory, cognition, and daily functioning. It's a progressive condition, and its risk increases with age. While there's no cure, early diagnosis, cognitive exercises, a balanced diet, and a stimulating environment can slow down its progression and enhance the quality of life for affected individuals.

6. Respiratory Disorders:
Chronic obstructive pulmonary disease (COPD), pneumonia, and other respiratory conditions are more common among seniors. Smoking, exposure to pollutants, and respiratory infections contribute to these disorders. Managing symptoms through medications, oxygen therapy, and pulmonary rehabilitation can improve quality of life for seniors with respiratory issues.

7. Cancer:
Cancer risk rises with age, and common types in seniors include lung, colorectal, breast, and prostate cancer. Early detection through screenings, healthy lifestyle choices, and advances in medical treatments have significantly improved cancer

outcomes. Regular screenings and adopting a healthy lifestyle can reduce the risk of cancer.

8. Depression and Anxiety:

Mental health issues such as depression and anxiety affect a significant number of seniors. Loss of loved ones, health problems, and social isolation can contribute to these conditions. Proper diagnosis, counseling, support groups, and social engagement are vital for managing mental health concerns in seniors.

9. Vision and Hearing Impairments:

Age-related vision and hearing loss are common issues in seniors. Conditions like cataracts, glaucoma, and macular degeneration affect vision, while hearing loss can result from exposure to noise, genetics, or age-related changes. Regular eye and hearing exams are essential for early detection and appropriate interventions.

10. Obesity:

Obesity, often linked to poor diet and lack of physical activity, can exacerbate various health issues in seniors, including diabetes, heart disease, and joint problems. Adopting a balanced diet and engaging in regular physical activity are crucial for managing weight and overall health.

Understanding these common health issues is the first step toward effective prevention, management, and improved quality of life for seniors. Regular medical check-ups, a healthy lifestyle, social engagement, and support from caregivers and healthcare professionals play pivotal roles in ensuring the well-being of the aging population.

How chair yoga can address health concerns

Chair yoga is a gentle and adaptable form of exercise that offers numerous benefits for seniors, addressing many of the health concerns commonly faced by this demographic. Through its combination of seated and standing poses, breathing exercises, and relaxation techniques, chair yoga provides a holistic approach to managing various health issues. Here's how chair yoga can address some of the most common health concerns in seniors:

1. Cardiovascular Health:
Chair yoga incorporates gentle cardiovascular exercises that elevate the heart rate and improve circulation. Poses like seated marching and seated jumping jacks, when practiced regularly, enhance cardiovascular health. Additionally, deep breathing exercises in chair yoga promote relaxation and help

regulate blood pressure, contributing to a healthier heart.

2. Arthritis and Joint Pain:
Chair yoga's gentle movements and stretches are excellent for improving joint flexibility and reducing arthritis pain. Seniors can engage in modified yoga poses that focus on the affected joints, helping to increase their range of motion. The controlled movements in chair yoga avoid stressing the joints while enhancing their mobility, making it an ideal practice for those with arthritis.

3. Osteoporosis:
Weight-bearing exercises are essential for individuals with osteoporosis to strengthen bones and reduce the risk of fractures. Chair yoga includes poses that target weight-bearing areas like the hips and spine, enhancing bone density and promoting bone health. These exercises, coupled with proper breathing techniques, aid in maintaining strong and healthy bones.

4. Diabetes Management:
Chair yoga supports diabetes management through gentle movements that improve circulation and promote insulin sensitivity. Regular practice helps regulate blood sugar levels. Additionally, chair yoga's relaxation techniques reduce stress, which is

beneficial for diabetes management, as stress can impact blood sugar levels.

5. Cognitive Health:

Chair yoga includes mindfulness practices and breathing exercises that enhance mental clarity and concentration. Engaging in these activities regularly supports cognitive function and can be particularly helpful for seniors dealing with dementia or Alzheimer's disease. The practice of chair yoga encourages focus, helping seniors maintain mental acuity.

6. Respiratory Health:

Chair yoga incorporates deep breathing exercises, which enhance lung capacity and improve respiratory function. Seniors with respiratory conditions like COPD benefit from these exercises, as they help in clearing the lungs and promoting better airflow. Enhanced breathing techniques also reduce anxiety and promote relaxation, contributing to overall respiratory well-being.

7. Depression and Anxiety:

Chair yoga's emphasis on mindfulness, meditation, and relaxation techniques helps reduce symptoms of depression and anxiety. Seniors practicing chair yoga experience a sense of calm and peace, which positively impacts their mental and emotional well-being. Regular participation in chair yoga classes also provides social interaction, reducing feelings of isolation and loneliness.

8. Vision and Hearing Impairments:
Chair yoga focuses on body awareness and does not rely heavily on visual cues, making it accessible for seniors with vision impairments. Instructors can use verbal cues and gentle touch to guide participants. Similarly, chair yoga classes can be adapted to accommodate seniors with hearing impairments, ensuring they can follow the exercises comfortably.

In conclusion, chair yoga serves as a versatile and inclusive solution to address the health concerns of seniors. Its gentle yet effective approach supports physical, mental, and emotional well-being. By practicing chair yoga regularly, seniors can enjoy improved flexibility, enhanced cardiovascular health, reduced pain, better bone density, enhanced cognitive function, and reduced symptoms of depression and anxiety. This accessible and beneficial practice empowers seniors to maintain their health, vitality, and overall quality of life.

Importance of flexibility, balance, and mental well-being in seniors

As individuals age, maintaining good health becomes increasingly essential to ensure a high quality of life. Three key components play a crucial role in senior well-being: flexibility, balance, and mental well-being. These elements are interconnected and contribute significantly to the overall health and vitality of seniors. Here is a detailed analysis of their significance:

1. Flexibility:

Flexibility is the term used to describe the range of motion in your joints and muscles. It's essential for seniors for several reasons:

- **Improved Mobility:** Flexible joints and muscles enable seniors to move more freely, making everyday activities easier and reducing the risk of injuries. Being able to bend, stretch, and twist comfortably is vital for maintaining independence in daily tasks.
- **Pain Prevention:** Flexible muscles and joints are less likely to become stiff or strained. Seniors with good flexibility experience fewer aches and pains, allowing

them to engage in activities without discomfort.

- **Enhanced Posture:** Good flexibility supports proper posture, reducing the risk of back pain and promoting spinal health. Seniors with flexible muscles can maintain an upright posture, which is essential for balance and overall well-being.
- **Maintaining Independence:** Seniors with good flexibility can perform activities such as reaching, bending, and dressing independently. This independence contributes to a positive self-image and overall confidence.

2. Balance:

Balance refers to the ability to control and stabilize the body during various movements and activities.

- **Fall Prevention:** Balance training is crucial for seniors as it significantly reduces the risk of falls. Falls are a leading cause of injuries among the elderly, often leading to fractures and loss of independence. Improving balance helps seniors maintain stability and prevent accidents.
- **Enhanced Mobility:** Good balance allows seniors to move with confidence and ease. It enables them to walk on uneven surfaces, navigate stairs, and engage in activities that

require controlled movements, promoting an active lifestyle.

- **Muscle Strength:** Balance exercises often engage various muscle groups, leading to improved muscle strength. Strong leg muscles, in particular, are essential for stability, supporting seniors in maintaining balance and preventing falls.
- **Cognitive Benefits:** Balance exercises challenge the brain and improve cognitive functions. Seniors who regularly engage in activities that challenge balance experience enhanced mental agility and better focus.

3. Mental Well-being:

Mental well-being encompasses emotional, psychological, and social aspects of health.

- **Reduced Stress:** Engaging in activities like yoga and meditation, which promote mental well-being, helps seniors manage stress. Chronic stress can contribute to various health issues, making relaxation techniques crucial for overall well-being.
- **Improved Mood:** Physical activity, including chair yoga, releases endorphins, which are known as "feel-good" hormones. Seniors who stay active and engaged often report improved mood, reduced feelings of depression, and increased overall happiness.

- **Enhanced Cognitive Function:** Regular mental stimulation, such as through puzzles, games, or learning new skills, supports brain health. Seniors who keep their minds active have a lower risk of cognitive decline and are better equipped to handle challenges.
- **Social Connection:** Maintaining social connections is vital for mental well-being. Seniors who participate in group activities, like chair yoga classes, have the opportunity to socialize, make new friends, and combat feelings of loneliness and isolation.

In summary, flexibility, balance, and mental well-being are integral components of senior health. Regular exercise, such as chair yoga, combined with activities that challenge the mind and promote relaxation, supports seniors in maintaining physical and mental vitality. By emphasizing these aspects of well-being, seniors can lead active, fulfilling lives and age gracefully while enjoying an excellent quality of life.

Chapter 3

Getting Started with Chair Yoga

Choosing the right chair and space for practicing

When it comes to practicing chair yoga, selecting the right chair and creating an appropriate space are essential steps that significantly impact the effectiveness and safety of your practice. Here's a detailed guide on how to choose the right chair and set up an ideal space for practicing chair yoga:

1. Choosing the Right Chair:
- **Sturdy and Stable:** Choose a chair that is sturdy and stable. Avoid chairs with wheels or that are too soft, as they can be unstable during certain yoga poses. A chair with four solid legs and a firm seat provides the necessary support for your practice.
- **Proper Height:** The chair should allow your feet to rest flat on the ground when you're

seated. Your knees should form a right angle, and your thighs should be parallel to the ground. This ensures proper alignment and comfort during the practice.

- **Armrests:** While not mandatory, chairs with armrests can provide additional support, especially for balance poses. However, make sure the armrests do not restrict your movement.

- **Comfortable Seat:** Choose a chair with a comfortable, flat seat. Padded seats can provide extra cushioning, making the practice more comfortable, especially if you plan on practicing for an extended period.

- **Backrest:** A chair with a straight backrest is preferable, as it supports good posture. However, some practitioners prefer chairs with a slight recline for relaxation poses. Select the choice that gives you the most comfort.

- **Adjustability (Optional):** If you have specific mobility concerns, consider chairs with adjustable height or removable armrests to accommodate your needs. Adjustable features allow for a customized and comfortable practice.

2. Creating the Ideal Space:

- **Ample Space:** Choose a room or area with enough space to move your arms and legs freely. Clear the space of any obstacles or furniture that could obstruct your movements during the practice. Having ample space ensures your safety and allows you to fully engage in the yoga poses.
- **Quiet Environment:** Select a quiet space where you can practice without disturbances. Eliminate noise and distractions, allowing you to focus on your breathing, movements, and relaxation. A serene environment enhances the overall yoga experience.
- **Good Lighting:** Natural light or well-lit spaces are ideal for practicing chair yoga. Proper lighting allows you to see your movements clearly, ensuring you maintain correct posture and alignment throughout the practice. If practicing in the evening or early morning, use soft, ambient lighting to create a calming atmosphere.
- **Ventilation:** Ensure the space is well-ventilated. Proper airflow is essential, especially if you are engaging in deep breathing exercises. Fresh air contributes to a comfortable and invigorating practice environment.

- **Personal Touch:** Consider adding personal touches to your practice space, such as calming colors, inspirational quotes, or soothing decor. These elements create a peaceful atmosphere, enhancing your overall yoga experience and promoting relaxation.

By carefully choosing the right chair and creating a suitable space for practicing chair yoga, you set the foundation for a safe, comfortable, and enjoyable practice. Remember, your practice space is your sanctuary, where you can focus on your well-being and embrace the benefits of chair yoga fully

Warm-up exercises tailored for seniors

Warm-up exercises are essential for seniors before engaging in any physical activity, including chair yoga. A proper warm-up routine helps increase blood flow to the muscles, prepares the body for movement, and reduces the risk of injuries. When tailored specifically for seniors, warm-up exercises focus on gentle movements that improve flexibility, enhance circulation, and promote joint mobility. Here's a detailed guide to warm-up exercises designed to benefit seniors:

1. Neck Stretches:

- **Neck Tilts:** Sit comfortably in your chair and slowly tilt your head to one side, bringing your ear toward your shoulder. Hold for a brief period of time before alternating sides.. Repeat this movement 3-5 times on each side to stretch the neck muscles gently.

Roll your neck gently in a clockwise and anticlockwise direction. Avoid quick or jerky movements to prevent strain. Neck rolls help release tension in the neck and improve range of motion.

2. Shoulder Rolls:

- **Forward Rolls:** Sit tall with your arms relaxed at your sides. Slowly roll your shoulders forward in a circle. Complete 10-15 rolls, then reverse the motion. Shoulder rolls ease tension in the upper back and shoulders, promoting flexibility and mobility.

3. Arm and Wrist Exercises:

- **Wrist Circles:** Extend your arms in front of you at shoulder height. Make gentle circles with your wrists, first clockwise, then counterclockwise. This exercise improves wrist flexibility and reduces stiffness.
- **Arm Raises:** Extend your arms straight overhead, then lower them back down. Repeat this motion 8-10 times. Arm raises

enhance shoulder mobility and increase blood flow to the upper body.

4. Spinal Twists:

- **Sitting Spinal Twist:** Place your feet flat on the floor while sitting tall in your chair. Place your right hand on your left knee and gently twist your torso to the left. Hold for a short while, then alternate sides. Spinal twists improve flexibility in the spine and promote a healthy range of motion.

5. Hip and Knee Flexibility:

- **Seated Marching:** Sit with your feet flat on the ground. Lift your right knee toward your chest, then lower it and lift the left knee. Continue this marching motion for 1-2 minutes. Seated marching improves hip and knee flexibility while engaging the leg muscles.
- **Ankle Rolls:** Lift one foot off the ground and rotate your ankle in a circular motion, first clockwise, then counterclockwise. Perform 10-15 rotations, then switch to the other foot. Ankle rolls enhance ankle mobility and reduce stiffness.

6. Breathing Exercises:

Sit comfortably and take a few deep breaths through your nose to fill your lungs with air. Exhale slowly through your mouth. Repeat this deep breathing exercise 5-10 times. Deep breathing increases oxygen flow to the muscles and calms the mind, preparing you for the yoga practice.

7. Mindfulness and Relaxation:
- **Body Scan:** Close your eyes and focus on each part of your body, starting from your toes and moving upward. Any regions that are tense or uncomfortable should be consciously relaxed. The body scan promotes relaxation and mental awareness, preparing your mind for the yoga practice.

When performing warm-up exercises, seniors should move slowly and gently, avoiding any sudden or jerky movements. Observe your body's signals and cease any motion that makes you feel pain or discomfort. By incorporating these tailored warm-up exercises into their routine, seniors can prepare their bodies and minds for chair yoga, ensuring a safe and enjoyable practice experience.

Breathing techniques for relaxation and focus

Breathing is a fundamental aspect of our existence, but it can also be a powerful tool for relaxation and focus. By incorporating specific breathing techniques into your routine, you can manage stress, enhance concentration, and promote overall well-being. Here's a comprehensive guide to various breathing techniques designed to help you relax and improve your focus:

1. Deep Abdominal Breathing:

Deep abdominal breathing, also known as diaphragmatic breathing, involves breathing deeply into your lungs, allowing your diaphragm to fully expand. This method encourages relaxation and lowers tension.

How to Practice:

Choose a comfortable position to sit or to lie down.

Your chest and abdomen should be touched with one hand each.

Inhale deeply through your nose, allowing your abdomen to expand as you fill your lungs with air.

As you slowly exhale out of your mouth, your stomach should contract.

Focus on the rise and fall of your abdomen with each breath, ensuring your chest remains relatively still.

Practice for 5-10 minutes, gradually extending the duration as you become more comfortable.

2. 4-7-8 Breathing:

The 4-7-8 breathing technique is a simple and effective method to promote relaxation and alleviate anxiety. It helps calm the nervous system, making it easier to focus and unwind.

How to Practice:

For a count of four, quietly inhale through your nose while closing your mouth.

Keep your breath held for seven counts.

For a count of eight, thoroughly and audibly exhale from your mouth.

This completes one breath cycle.

Repeat this cycle for 4 breaths initially, gradually increasing the repetitions as you become accustomed to the technique.

3. Alternate Nostril Breathing (Nadi Shodhana):

This ancient yogic breathing technique balances the two hemispheres of the brain, promoting mental clarity, focus, and relaxation.

How to Practice:

Set your spine in a neutral position and find a nice seat.

Use your right thumb to cover your right nostril and take a deep breath through your left nose.

After inhaling, close your left nostril with your right ring finger, releasing your right nostril.

Exhale completely through your right nostril.

Inhale deeply through your right nostril, then close it with your right thumb.

Release your left nostril and exhale completely through your left nostril.

This completes one cycle.

Repeat for 5-10 cycles, focusing on your breath and maintaining a calm rhythm.

4. Belly Breathing with Counting:

Combining deep abdominal breathing with counting helps regulate your breath and enhances your focus and relaxation.

How to Practice:

Your chest and abdomen should be touched with one hand each.

Inhale slowly and deeply through your nose, expanding your abdomen. Count silently to 4 during the inhalation.

Exhale slowly and completely through your mouth, contracting your abdomen. Count silently to 4 during the exhalation.

Continue this pattern, inhaling and exhaling for a count of 4 each, ensuring your breaths are deep and steady.

Focus on the counting and the rise and fall of your abdomen, clearing your mind of distractions.

5. Box Breathing (Square Breathing):

Box breathing is a rhythmic technique that helps balance your nervous system, reducing stress and promoting relaxation and focus.

How to Practice:

Inhale through your nose for four counts.

For four counts, hold your breath.

For a count of four, completely exhale through your mouth.

Pause and hold your breath for another count of 4 before inhaling again.

For several rounds, repeat this pattern, progressively lengthening each count as you gain comfort.

6. Guided Visualization Breathing:

Guided visualization breathing combines deep breathing with mental imagery, allowing you to visualize calming scenes or experiences. This technique enhances relaxation and focus by engaging your senses and imagination.

How to Practice:

To unwind, close your eyes and take a few slow, deep breaths.

Inhale deeply and imagine a peaceful place, such as a beach, forest, or garden. Visualize the details, colors, and textures of the scene.

As you exhale, imagine releasing any tension or stress, allowing it to dissolve into the surroundings of your chosen visualization.

Continue to inhale positive energy and exhale negativity, immersing yourself in the calming imagery.

Practice this technique for 5-10 minutes, allowing your mind to fully engage with the guided visualization.

7. Ujjayi Breathing:

Ujjayi breathing, also known as ocean breath, is a yogic breathing technique that involves slightly constricting the back of your throat, creating a subtle sound resembling ocean waves. This technique promotes relaxation, focus, and mindfulness.

How to Practice:

Maintain a straight back and relaxed shoulders while you sit.

Inhale deeply through your nose while slightly constricting the back of your throat, creating a soft hissing sound in the back of your throat.

Exhale slowly and audibly through your nose while maintaining the same throat constriction, producing a gentle, soothing sound

Focus on the rhythmic sound of your breath, allowing it to calm your mind and deepen your concentration.

Practice this technique for 5-10 minutes, adjusting the pace of your breath to match your comfort level.

Each of these breathing techniques offers unique benefits for relaxation and focus. Incorporate them into your daily routine, especially before or after your yoga practice, meditation, or during stressful situations. By mastering these techniques, you can enhance your overall well-being, reduce anxiety, and improve your ability to concentrate, leading to a more peaceful and focused state of mind

Chapter 4

Chair Yoga Poses for Mobility and Flexibility

Seated yoga poses to improve joint flexibility

Seated yoga poses offer a gentle yet effective way to enhance joint flexibility, especially for individuals who may have limited mobility or prefer a practice with minimal impact. These poses focus on stretching and mobilizing various joints in the body, promoting increased flexibility and ease of movement. Here's a comprehensive guide to seated yoga poses designed to improve joint flexibility:

1. Seated Neck Stretches:
- **Neck Tilt:** Sit comfortably with a straight back. Bring your ear towards your shoulder as you slowly incline your head to one side. Hold for a few breaths, feeling the stretch in your neck. Repeat on the other side.

- **Neck Rotation:** Turn your head to the right as far as comfortable, holding for a few breaths. Repeat on the left side after coming back to the centre. . This stretch improves neck flexibility and reduces stiffness.

2. Seated Shoulder Stretches:

- **Shoulder Rolls:** Sit tall with your hands resting on your knees. Roll your shoulders in a circle forward, then do the opposite. Shoulder rolls release tension in the shoulders and improve mobility.
- **Eagle Arms:** Extend your arms in front of you, then cross your right arm over the left. Bend your elbows and bring your palms together, if possible. Lift your elbows slightly, feeling a stretch between your shoulder blades. Change sides after a few breaths of holding.

3. Seated Spinal Twists:
- **Simple Spinal Twist:** Sit with your legs crossed. Put your left hand behind you and your right hand on your left knee. Inhale to lengthen your spine, then exhale and twist to the left. Hold for a few breaths, feeling the twist in your spine. Repeat on the other side.

- **Half Lord of the Fishes Pose (Ardha Matsyendrasana):** Sit with your legs extended. Place your foot outside of your left thigh while bending your right knee. Cross your left elbow over your right knee and twist to the right. Change sides after a few breaths of holding. This position increases spinal mobility and flexibility.

4. Seated Hip Stretches:

- **Seated Forward Bend:** Sit with your legs extended. Inhale to lengthen your spine, then exhale and hinge at your hips, reaching your hands toward your feet. Hold for a few breaths, feeling the stretch in your hamstrings and lower back.
- **Butterfly Pose (Baddha Konasana):** Sit with your legs bent and the soles of your feet together. Hold your feet and gently press your knees toward the floor. Sit tall and breathe deeply, feeling the stretch in your inner thighs and hips.

5. Seated Knee and Ankle Stretches:
- **Seated Knee Extension:** Sit with your legs extended. Right knee bent; bring heel of right foot close to torso. Hold your shin or use a strap around your foot for support.

Change sides after a few breaths of holding. This stretch improves knee flexibility.

- **Ankle Circles:** Extend your legs and lift your feet off the ground. Rotate your ankles in circular motions, first clockwise, then counterclockwise. This movement enhances ankle mobility and reduces stiffness.

6. Seated Wrist and Hand Stretches:

- **Wrist Circles:** Extend your arms in front of you. Rotate your wrists in circular motions, first clockwise, then counterclockwise. This stretch improves wrist flexibility and reduces tension.
- **Finger Stretch:** Extend your right arm forward, palm facing down. Use your left hand to gently press your fingers toward the floor, feeling a stretch in your forearm and fingers. Change sides after a few breaths of holding.

7. Seated Ankle-to-Knee Stretch:

- **Seated Ankle-to-Knee Pose (Agastya Parivrtta Sukhasana):** Sit with your right knee bent and your right foot placed on your left thigh. Inhale to lengthen your spine, then exhale and twist to the right, placing your left elbow outside your right knee. Change sides after a few breaths of holding.

This pose stretches the hips and improves spinal flexibility.

8. Seated Cat-Cow Stretch:

- **Seated Cat-Cow Pose:** Sit with your hands resting on your knees. Inhale and arch your back (cow pose), lifting your chest and chin. Take a breath out, round your back, and tuck your chin into your chest (the cat stance). Repeat this movement for a few rounds, synchronizing your breath with the motion. This stretch enhances spinal flexibility and mobility.

When practicing seated yoga poses to improve joint flexibility, focus on gentle and controlled movements. Never force yourself into a stretch, and listen to your body's signals. Incorporate deep breathing and mindful awareness into your practice to enhance the overall benefits. With consistent practice, these seated yoga poses can significantly enhance joint flexibility, reduce stiffness, and promote overall mobility and well-being.

Gentle stretches to increase mobility

Mobility is essential for maintaining independence and overall well-being, especially as we age. Gentle stretches play a vital role in enhancing flexibility, improving joint range of motion, and promoting ease of movement. These stretches focus on gentle and controlled movements, making them accessible to individuals with various fitness levels and mobility challenges. Here's a comprehensive guide to gentle stretches designed to increase mobility and promote flexibility:

1. Neck and Shoulder Stretches:
- **Neck Tilt:** Sit or stand comfortably. Bring your ear towards your shoulder as you slowly incline your head to one side. Hold for a few seconds, feeling the stretch in your neck. Repeat on the opposite side after returning to the centre.
- **Shoulder Rolls:** Circularly roll your shoulders forward, then the other way. This movement helps release tension in the shoulders and improves mobility.

2. Chest Opener:
- **Standing or Seated Chest Opener:** Stand tall or sit with a straight back. Clasp your hands behind your back and gently straighten your arms while lifting your chest. Hold for a few breaths, feeling the stretch across your chest and shoulders. This stretch improves posture and opens the chest area.

3. Spinal Twist:

- **Seated Spinal Twist:** Sit with your legs crossed. Put your left hand behind you and your right hand on your left knee. Inhale to lengthen your spine, then exhale and twist to the left. Hold for a few breaths, feeling the stretch in your spine. Repeat on the other side.

4. Hip Flexor Stretch:

Sit on the edge of a chair and perform a seated hip flexor stretch. Extend your right leg straight and bend your left knee, placing your left foot flat on the ground. Feel your right hip flexor being stretched as you gently lean forward. Change sides after a few breaths of holding.

5. Quadriceps Stretch:

- **Standing Quadriceps Stretch:** Stand near a wall or a sturdy surface for balance. Hold onto the wall with your left hand. Bring your right heel up towards your buttocks while bending your right knee. Grab your right ankle with your right hand and gently pull, feeling the stretch in your quadriceps. Change sides after a few breaths of holding.

6. Hamstring Stretch:

- **Seated Hamstring Stretch:** Sit on the floor with your legs extended straight. Inhale to lengthen your spine, then exhale and reach forward toward your toes. According on your level of flexibility, hold onto your shins, ankles, or feet. Hold the stretch for a few breaths, feeling the stretch in your hamstrings and lower back.

7. Calf Stretch:

- **Calf Stretch:** Stand facing a wall. Place your hands against the wall at shoulder height. Step your right foot back and press your heel down toward the floor. Keep your back leg straight and feel the stretch in your calf. Change sides after a few breaths of holding.

8. Ankle Mobility Exercise:

- **Ankle Circles:** Sit or stand comfortably. Lift one foot off the ground and rotate your ankle in circular motions, first clockwise, then counterclockwise. Perform 10-15 rotations, then switch to the other foot. This movement enhances ankle mobility and reduces stiffness.

9. Wrist and Forearm Stretch:

- **Wrist Stretch:** Extend your right arm forward, palm facing down. Use your left hand to gently press your fingers toward the floor, feeling a stretch in your wrist and forearm. Change sides after a few breaths of holding.

10. Deep Breathing with Arm Movements:

- **Deep Breathing with Arm Raises:** Inhale deeply through your nose while raising your arms overhead. Exhale slowly through your mouth while lowering your arms. Focus on your breath and the gentle movement of your arms. This exercise promotes relaxation and enhances mobility in the shoulder joints.

Tips for Safe Stretching:

- **Warm Up:** Perform light aerobic exercises or gentle movements to warm up your body before stretching.
- **Gentle Movements:** Move slowly and avoid jerky or sudden movements, especially if you have joint issues.
- Pay attention to your body and simply stretch until you experience slight discomfort, not pain.
- **Consistency:** Incorporate these stretches into your daily routine to improve mobility gradually.

- **Breathing:** Breathe deeply and rhythmically during each stretch to enhance relaxation and flexibility.

Incorporating these gentle stretches into your daily routine can significantly improve your mobility, flexibility, and overall well-being. Remember, consistency and patience are key when working on increasing your mobility. With regular practice, you'll notice improvements in your range of motion and feel more comfortable in your daily movements.

Modifications for different fitness levels

Fitness is a personal journey, and every individual's capabilities and needs are unique. Inclusive fitness practices embrace the diversity of abilities, ensuring that people of all fitness levels can participate and benefit. Here's a detailed guide on modifications tailored for different fitness levels, promoting inclusivity and enabling everyone to engage in physical activities:

1. Beginners:

- **Slow Pacing:** Beginners should start with slow and controlled movements to build a foundation of strength and stability. Place more emphasis on technique and perfect form than on speed.

- **Light Resistance:** Use lighter weights or resistance bands to avoid strain. Gradually increase resistance as strength and endurance improve.
- **Rest and Recovery:** Allow sufficient rest between exercises and workouts. Adequate rest promotes muscle recovery and reduces the risk of injuries.
- **Simplified Movements:** Choose simplified versions of exercises. For example, perform modified push-ups with knees on the ground before progressing to full push-ups.

2. Intermediate Participants:

- **Moderate Intensity:** Intermediate participants can engage in moderate-intensity workouts that challenge their endurance and strength. Increase the pace and intensity of exercises while maintaining proper form.
- **Diverse Workouts:** Incorporate a variety of exercises, including cardio, strength training, and flexibility exercises. Diversifying the workout routine ensures overall fitness and prevents plateauing.
- **Heavier Weights:** Gradually increase the weight or resistance to challenge muscle

strength. Use heavier dumbbells or resistance bands to promote muscle growth and endurance.

- **Interval Training:** Introduce interval training, alternating between periods of high-intensity exercises and active recovery. This approach boosts cardiovascular fitness and burns more calories.

3. Advanced Athletes:

- **High Intensity:** Advanced athletes can engage in high-intensity workouts, including HIIT (High-Intensity Interval Training) and advanced cardio exercises. These workouts elevate heart rate, burn calories, and improve endurance.
- **Progressive Overload:** Focus on progressive overload, gradually increasing resistance, duration, or intensity to continue challenging the body. Progressive overload is essential for muscle and strength gains.
- **Compound Movements:** Incorporate complex, multi-joint exercises like squats, deadlifts, and bench presses. Compound movements engage multiple muscle groups, promoting overall strength and muscle coordination.
- **Incorporate Challenges:** Add challenges such as plyometric exercises, agility drills,

or advanced yoga poses to enhance balance, coordination, and athletic performance.

4. Modifications for Seniors:

- **Low-Impact Exercises:** Opt for low-impact exercises to protect joints and reduce the risk of injuries. Activities like walking, swimming, or chair exercises are gentle on the joints.
- **Chair Modifications:** For individuals with limited mobility or balance issues, chair exercises are highly effective. Seated marches, seated leg lifts, and seated torso twists can be performed comfortably.
- **Focus on Flexibility:** Include regular stretching exercises to improve flexibility and maintain joint mobility. Yoga and tai chi are excellent choices for seniors, promoting balance, flexibility, and relaxation.
- **Light Resistance:** Seniors can use light resistance bands or light dumbbells for strength training. Focus on higher repetitions and proper form to build muscle endurance.

5. Modifications for Individuals with Disabilities:

- **Adapted Equipment:** Use adapted equipment such as resistance bands with handles, stability balls, or modified weight machines designed for individuals with disabilities.

- **Seated Exercises:** Many exercises can be modified to seated positions, allowing individuals with limited mobility or wheelchair users to engage in strength and flexibility training.
- **Assisted Movements:** Involve assistance devices or support from caregivers or trainers to perform exercises safely. For example, using parallel bars for balance or having a spotter during weightlifting.
- **Tailored Programs:** Seek the guidance of fitness professionals experienced in adaptive fitness. They can design personalized workout programs that cater to specific disabilities and abilities, ensuring safe and effective exercises.

Incorporating these modifications for different fitness levels ensures that fitness routines are inclusive and accessible to everyone. Whether you're a beginner starting your fitness journey, an intermediate participant looking to challenge yourself, an advanced athlete aiming for peak performance, a senior focusing on mobility, or an individual with disabilities seeking adaptive fitness, these modifications empower individuals to embrace physical activity and improve their overall health and well-being. Remember, consistency, safety, and personalized guidance are key components of any successful fitness journey, regardless of your fitness level or abilities.

Chapter 5

Chair Yoga for Balance and Stability

Balancing poses to enhance stability

Balancing poses in yoga are not just about standing on one leg; they are a profound practice of stability, focus, and strength. Incorporating these poses into your fitness routine not only enhances physical stability but also cultivates mental balance and concentration. Here's a detailed guide to various balancing poses that can help enhance your stability and overall well-being:

1. Tree Pose (Vrksasana):
Tree Pose is a fundamental balancing pose that strengthens your legs and core muscles while improving stability and focus.
How to Practice:

Stand tall with your feet together. Shift your weight onto your left foot and place your right foot on your inner left thigh or calf (avoid the knee).

Bring your palms together in front of your chest or raise your arms overhead, reaching for the sky.

Focus on a fixed point in front of you to maintain balance. Switch sides after holding for a few breaths.

2. Warrior III (Virabhadrasana III):

Warrior III pose builds strength in your legs and core muscles while challenging your balance and stability.

How to Practice:

Standing upright with your feet hip-width apart is a good place to start.

Shift your weight onto your right foot, lift your left leg straight behind you, and parallel to the ground.

Reach your arms forward, creating a straight line from your hands to your left heel.

Keep your hips level and your body in one straight line. Switch sides after holding for a few breaths.

3. Eagle Pose (Garudasana):

Eagle Pose enhances balance, stability, and concentration while stretching and strengthening your legs and shoulders.

How to Practice:

Stand with your feet together. Cross your right thigh over your left thigh by slightly bending your knees. Hook your right foot around your left calf if possible. Cross your left arm over your right arm, bringing your palms together in front of your face.

Focus on a point in front of you and maintain balance. Switch sides after holding for a few breaths.

4. Half Moon Pose (Ardha Chandrasana):

Half Moon Pose improves balance, stability, and strengthens your legs, core, and hips.

How to Practice:

Begin in a standing position. Shift your weight onto your right foot and bring your left hand to the floor about a foot in front of your right foot.

Lift your left leg parallel to the ground and extend your right arm toward the sky. Stack your hips and shoulders.

Engage your core and gaze at your right hand. Switch sides after holding for a few breaths.

5. Extended Hand-to-Big-Toe Pose (Utthita Hasta Padangusthasana):

This pose challenges your balance and enhances stability in the standing leg while stretching your hamstrings.

How to Practice:

Stand tall and place your weight on your left foot. Lift your right leg in front of you and hold your big toe with your right hand. Straighten your leg.

If you cannot reach your toe, use a yoga strap around the sole of your foot for assistance.

Keep your left hand on your hip or extend it to the side for balance. Switch sides after holding for a few breaths.

6. Scale Pose (Tolasana):

Scale Pose is an arm balance that requires strong arms and core muscles while challenging your stability and balance.

How to Practice:

Sit with your legs crossed. Place your hands on the floor beside your hips, fingers pointing forward.

Press into your hands, engage your core, and lift your hips off the ground. Straighten your arms and keep your legs lifted.

Hold the pose for a few breaths, focusing on engaging your core muscles. Gently lower down and repeat.

7. Garland Pose (Malasana):

Garland Pose strengthens your ankles, thighs, and core muscles while enhancing stability and flexibility.

How to Practice:

As you stand, your feet should be roughly hip-width apart. Lower your body into a squat position, keeping your heels on the ground.

While pressing your legs outward with your elbows, bring your palms together at your heart's centre.

Keep your spine straight and chest lifted. Hold the position for a few breaths while noticing how your hips and thighs are stretched.

8. One-Legged King Pigeon Pose (Eka Pada Rajakapotasana):

This advanced yoga pose improves balance, hip flexibility, and stability while opening the chest and shoulders.

How to Practice:

Start in a downward-facing dog position. Bring your right knee toward your chest and slide your foot forward, placing it between your hands.

Untuck your toes and bring your left knee to the floor. As you take a breath, elevate your chest and arch your back.

Reach your right hand back and grab your left foot, bringing it toward your head. Switch sides after holding for a few breaths.

Tips for Balancing Poses:
- **Focus and Concentration:** Concentrate on a fixed point (a "drishti") to help maintain balance and stability.

- **Engage Core Muscles:** Strong core muscles provide stability. Engage your abdominal muscles to support your balance.
- **Start with Support:** Use a wall, chair, or yoga block for support while practicing balancing poses. Gradually reduce support as your stability improves.
- **Breathe Mindfully:** Focus on your breath to calm your mind and enhance your focus. Smooth and steady breathing aids in balance.
- **Practice Regularly:** Consistent practice is key to improving stability. Include balancing poses in your routine regularly to build strength and stability over time.

Balancing poses are not just physical exercises; they are opportunities to cultivate mindfulness, concentration, and inner stability. With patience, practice, and mindful breathing, these poses can transform not only your physical balance but also your mental and emotional equilibrium, leading to a more centered and grounded you.

Techniques to improve posture and core strength

Good posture and core strength are essential components of overall physical health. They not only contribute to a confident and poised appearance but also support a healthy spine, prevent back pain, and enhance overall body stability. Here's a detailed guide to techniques that can help you improve your posture and strengthen your core muscles effectively:

1. Posture Improvement Techniques:
a. Awareness and Mindfulness:
- **Body Scan:** Regularly scan your body from head to toe, noticing any areas of tension or discomfort. The first step in posture improvement is awareness.
- **Mirror Check:** Use a mirror to observe your posture from the side. Check for a straight line from your earlobe through your shoulder, hip, knee, and ankle. Make adjustments as needed.

b. Ergonomics and Workspace Setup:
- **Chair and Desk Height:** Adjust your chair and desk to the appropriate height so your feet are flat on the floor, and your knees and hips are at 90-degree angles. To support your lower back's natural curve, use a cushion or lumbar roll.
- **Screen Level:** Position your computer screen at eye level to avoid tilting your head up or down. This prevents strain on your neck and upper back.

c. Strengthening Exercises:

- **Upper Back Exercises:** Perform exercises like rows and shoulder squeezes to strengthen the upper back muscles, improving posture and preventing slouching.

- **Neck Stretches:** Gently stretch your neck muscles by tilting your head from side to side and forward and backward. Hold each stretch for a few seconds to release tension.

- **Wall Angels:** Stand with your back against a wall and your arms in a goalpost position. Slide your arms up and down the wall, engaging your shoulder blades. This exercise promotes proper shoulder alignment.

d. Yoga and Pilates:

- **Cobra Pose (Bhujangasana):** Lie on your stomach, place your hands under your shoulders, and lift your chest while keeping your pelvis on the ground. Cobra pose strengthens the lower back and promotes a healthy spine.

- **Pilates Roll-Up:** Lie on your back, extend your arms overhead, and roll up, reaching for your toes. This exercise engages your core muscles and improves spinal flexibility.

e. Corrective Devices:

- **Posture Correctors:** Consider using posture correctors, especially during desk work or prolonged periods of sitting. These devices provide gentle support to help maintain an upright posture.

- **Orthopaedic Chairs:** Invest in an ergonomic chair designed to support proper posture. These chairs provide lumbar support and encourage a natural spine alignment.

2. Core Strengthening Techniques:
a. Basic Core Exercises:

- Starting in a push-up position with your arms straight, perform a plank. Using your core muscles, maintain a straight line from your head to your heels. Hold the plank for as long as you can, gradually increasing the duration.
- **Russian Twists:** Kneel down on the ground with your heels flat on the ground. Lean back slightly and twist your torso to the right, then to the left, tapping the ground beside your hip. This exercise targets the oblique muscles.
- **Bird Dogs:** Kneel on your hands and knees. Extend your right arm forward and your left leg backward, keeping your back flat. Switch sides after a brief period of holding. Bird dogs strengthen the lower back and core muscles.

b. Balance and Stability Exercises:

- **Bosu Ball Squats:** Stand on a Bosu ball (half stability ball) with your feet hip-width apart. Perform squats, engaging your core muscles for stability. The unstable surface challenges your balance and strengthens your core.
- **Single-Leg Stance:** Stand on one leg while keeping the other lifted slightly off the ground. Hold the position for as long as you can, then switch legs. This exercise enhances balance and core stability.

c. Dynamic Core Workouts:

- **Mountain Climbers:** Start in a push-up position. Running-like, alternately bring your knees to your chest. Mountain climbers engage your core, legs, and cardiovascular system simultaneously.
- **Plank Variations:** Try plank variations such as side planks, forearm planks, and plank leg lifts. These variations target different muscles within the core, enhancing overall strength and stability.

d. Cardiovascular Activities:

- **Swimming:** Swimming engages the entire body, including the core muscles, providing an excellent cardiovascular workout while strengthening your core.

- **Dance Workouts:** Dance-based workouts like Zumba or hip-hop dance engage the core muscles while offering a fun and energetic way to exercise.

e. Breathing and Core Activation:

- **Diaphragmatic Breathing:** Practice diaphragmatic breathing to engage your diaphragm and core muscles. Deeply inhale through your nose while allowing your stomach to swell. Exhale slowly through your mouth, pulling your navel toward your spine.
- **Core Activation Exercises:** Perform exercises that focus on activating the deep core muscles, such as pelvic tilts and abdominal hollowing. These exercises enhance core stability and support proper posture.

f. Functional Movements:

- **Squatting:** Practice proper squatting techniques, engaging your core muscles as you lower your body. Squats strengthen the core, legs, and glutes, promoting functional strength for daily activities.
- **Lifting Techniques:** When lifting objects, bend your knees, keep your back straight, and engage your core muscles. Proper lifting techniques protect your spine and enhance core strength.

Tips for Success:

- **Consistency:** Regularly practice these techniques to see noticeable improvements in posture and core strength.
- **Gradual Progression:** Start with beginner-level exercises and gradually progress to more challenging ones as your strength and stability improve.
- **Proper Form:** Focus on proper form and technique to maximize the effectiveness of each exercise and prevent injuries.
- **Mind-Body Connection:** Stay mindful of your body's movements and sensations. Mindful exercises enhance body awareness and improve posture.
- **Professional Guidance:** If you are unsure about the correct techniques, consider consulting a fitness trainer or physical therapist for personalized guidance and support.

By incorporating these techniques into your daily routine and fitness regimen, you can build a strong foundation of core strength and maintain excellent posture. Over time, these practices not only enhance your physical well-being but also boost your confidence, ensuring you stand tall and move with grace and ease. Remember, consistency, patience, and a mindful approach are key to achieving lasting improvements in posture and core strength.

Fall prevention exercises

Falls are a significant concern, especially for older adults, but the good news is that many falls can be prevented through regular exercise. Fall prevention exercises focus on improving balance, strength, flexibility, and coordination, reducing the risk of falls and enhancing overall stability. Here's a detailed guide to a variety of exercises designed to prevent falls and promote confidence in daily movements:

1. Balance Exercises:
a. Standing on One Leg:
Stand near a counter or sturdy chair for support.
Lift one foot slightly off the ground and balance on the other leg.
Hold the position for 10-30 seconds, then switch legs.
Increase the duration gradually as your balance gets better.
b. Heel-to-Toe Walk:
Walk in a straight line, placing the heel of one foot directly in front of the toes of the other foot each time you take a step.

Focus on a point ahead of you to maintain balance. Walk for 20 steps, then turn around and walk back.

c. Balance Exercises with Balance Disc or Wobble Board:

Stand on a balance disc or wobble board, engaging your core muscles to maintain stability.

Perform simple exercises like squats or arm raises while balancing on the unstable surface.

These tools challenge your balance and improve proprioception (awareness of body position).

2. Strength Exercises:

a. Bodyweight Squats:

Stand with your feet shoulder-width apart.

Lower your body as if you are sitting back into a chair, keeping your chest lifted and your knees aligned with your toes.

To return to your starting position, drive through your heels.

Aim for 2-3 sets of 10-15 repetitions.

b. Leg Raises:

Hold onto a sturdy surface like a chair or countertop for balance.

Lift one leg straight back without bending your knee.

Bring your leg back down after a brief holding period.

Do 2-3 sets of 10-15 repetitions on each leg.

c. Calf Raises:

Stand with your feet flat on the ground.

Lifting your torso onto the balls of your feet, slowly lift your heels off the ground.

Lower your heels back down.

Perform 2-3 sets of 15-20 repetitions.

3. Flexibility and Stretching Exercises:

a. Neck and Shoulder Stretches:

Gently tilt your head to the side, bringing your ear toward your shoulder to stretch your neck.

Shift your shoulders back and forth to de-stress.

Perform these stretches for 20-30 seconds on each side.

b. Hip and Quadriceps Stretches:

Stand near a chair for support.

Bend your knee and grab your ankle behind you with your hand.

Gently pull your ankle toward your buttocks, feeling a stretch in your quadriceps.

Hold for 20-30 seconds, then switch sides.

c. Hamstring and Calf Stretches:

The sole of your foot should be against the inside of your thigh when you sit on the floor with one leg extended straight ahead and the other leg bent.

Reach forward toward your toes, feeling a stretch in your hamstring.

Hold for 20-30 seconds, then switch legs.

For calf stretches, stand facing a wall and place one foot behind you, keeping your heel on the ground. Lean forward to feel the stretch in your calf.

4. Coordination and Agility Exercises:

a. Toe Taps:

Stand in front of a low step or platform.

Alternate tapping your toes on the step, moving quickly and lightly.

Aim for 2-3 sets of 30 seconds.

b. Ladder Drills:

Use an agility ladder or draw ladder patterns on the ground with chalk.

Practice stepping in and out of the ladder squares in various patterns, such as side steps, crossover steps, and high knees.

Perform ladder drills for 5-10 minutes, focusing on coordination and quick footwork.

c. Tai Chi or Yoga:

Participate in classes or follow instructional videos for Tai Chi or yoga, both of which emphasize balance, flexibility, and controlled movements.

These practices enhance body awareness and improve stability over time.

5. Vision and Sensory Integration Exercises:

a. Eye Tracking Exercises:

Sit or stand in a comfortable position.

Move your eyes from side to side, then up and down.

Without moving your head, follow a moving object with your eyes.

These exercises improve eye coordination and visual focus.

b. Sensory Integration Activities:

Walk barefoot on different surfaces like grass, sand, or textured mats.

Use sensory balls or balance pads to challenge your sense of touch and proprioception.

Engaging with various textures improves sensory feedback and enhances stability.

6. Regular Aerobic Exercises:

a. Walking:

Engage in brisk walking for at least 30 minutes a day, aiming for a total of 150 minutes of moderate aerobic activity per week.

Walking strengthens your legs, improves cardiovascular health, and enhances overall endurance.

b. Swimming:

Participate in water aerobics programmes or lap swimming.

Water provides resistance and supports your body, making it an excellent low-impact exercise for all fitness levels.

c. Dancing:

Take dance classes or follow dance workout videos at home.

Dancing improves coordination, balance, and cardiovascular fitness while having fun.

Tips for Fall Prevention Exercises:

- **Consult a Professional:** If you have existing health conditions or concerns, consult a healthcare provider or physical therapist before starting any exercise program.
- **Progress Gradually:** Start with exercises that match your current fitness level and gradually increase the intensity and duration over time.
- **Use Proper Footwear:** Wear supportive and well-fitted shoes, both indoors and outdoors, to prevent slips and falls.
- **Home Safety:** Keep your living space clutter-free, secure rugs and carpets to the floor, and install grab bars in bathrooms for additional safety.
- **Stay Hydrated:** Drink water regularly, especially during exercise, to prevent dizziness and dehydration, which can contribute to falls.

By incorporating these fall prevention exercises into your daily routine, you can significantly reduce the risk of falls, enhance your balance and coordination, and improve your overall confidence in movement. Remember that consistency and dedication are key to reaping the benefits of these exercises. Stay mindful of your body, focus on proper form, and enjoy the increased stability and well-being that these exercises can bring to your life.

Chapter 6

Chair Yoga for Pain Relief

Yoga poses to alleviate common pains

Yoga, an ancient practice that combines physical postures, breathing exercises, and meditation, offers a holistic approach to alleviate various common pains such as back pain, neck discomfort, and arthritis. By incorporating yoga into your daily routine, you can enhance flexibility, strengthen muscles, and improve overall well-being. Here's a comprehensive guide to yoga poses specifically designed to alleviate these common pains:

1. Back Pain:
a. Child's Pose (Balasana):
Kneel on the mat with your knees apart and your big toes touching.
Lowering your forehead to the ground while leaning back on your heels and reaching your arms forward.
Relax in this position, allowing your spine to lengthen and release tension in the lower back.

b. Cat-Cow Pose (Marjaryasana-Bitilasana):

Start by putting your hands and legs together in a tabletop position.

Taking a breath in, elevate your head and tailbone while arching your back (Cow Pose).

Take a breath out, arch your back, and chin-tuck into the "Cat Pose."

Flow between these positions, syncing your breath with the movements to massage and stretch your spine.

c. Downward-Facing Dog (Adho Mukha Svanasana):

Start on your hands and knees, then lift your hips toward the ceiling, straightening your legs.

Press your palms and heels into the ground, creating an inverted V shape with your body.

Downward Dog stretches the entire back, strengthening the spine and relieving back pain.

2. Neck Discomfort:

a. Neck Rolls:

Sit or stand with your spine straight.

Slowly drop your chin toward your chest and roll your head in a circular motion, moving clockwise and then counterclockwise.

Neck rolls release tension in the neck muscles and improve mobility.

b. Seated Neck Stretch:

Sit cross-legged with your spine tall.

Tilt your right ear toward your right shoulder, feeling a stretch along the left side of your neck.

Hold for a few breaths, then switch sides. Repeat as needed to alleviate neck discomfort.

c. Eagle Arms (Garudasana Arms):

Sit or stand comfortably.

Extend your arms forward, then cross your right arm over your left, bringing your palms to touch (or as close as possible).

Your upper back and shoulders will stretch when you lift your elbows just a little.

Hold for a few breaths, then switch the crossing of your arms.

3. Arthritis:

a. Supine Hand Stretch:

Knees bent and feet flat on the floor, lie on your back.

Extend your arms straight overhead, palms facing up.

Use your other hand to gently pull the fingers of one hand, stretching your wrists and fingers.

Hold for a few breaths, then switch hands.

b. Chair Pose (Utkatasana):

Put your feet together and keep your arms at your sides.

Inhale, raise your arms overhead, and bend your knees, as if sitting back into an imaginary chair.

Engage your thighs and core. Hold the pose, breathing deeply, to strengthen leg muscles and improve joint flexibility.

c. Supported Bridge Pose:

Knees bent and feet hip-width apart, lie on your back.

Place a block or cushion under your sacrum (lower back).

Relax in this supported position, allowing your hips and lower back to release tension.

Supported Bridge Pose gently stretches the spine and stimulates the abdominal organs.

4. Headaches:

a. Seated Forward Bend (Paschimottanasana):

Legs straight out in front of you when you sit.

Inhale, lengthen your spine, then exhale and fold forward from your hips, reaching for your feet or shins.

Relax your head and neck, allowing the weight of your head to release tension.

Paschimottanasana calms the mind and relieves stress, often contributing to headache relief.

b. Pose with the Legs Up the Wall (Viparita Karani):

Sit with your side against a wall, then gently swing your legs up the wall as you lie down.

Put your arms at your sides with the palms facing upward.

Close your eyes and focus on your breath. Relax in this inversion to reduce headaches and promote relaxation.

c. Child's Pose (Balasana):

Kneel on the mat with your knees apart and your big toes touching.

Lowering your forehead to the ground while leaning back on your heels and reaching your arms forward. Rest in Child's Pose, allowing your forehead to touch the mat and releasing any tension in your head and neck.

Tips for Practicing Yoga to Alleviate Pains:

- **Listen to Your Body:** Honor your body's limitations and avoid pushing yourself into discomfort or pain during yoga practice.
- **Warm-Up:** Begin with gentle warm-up exercises or stretches to prepare your body for deeper poses.
- **Breath Awareness:** Focus on deep, rhythmic breathing to relax your mind and enhance the effectiveness of the poses.
- **Regular Practice:** Consistency is key. Regular yoga practice, even for a few minutes daily, can provide significant relief from common pains.
- **Professional Guidance:** If you have specific health concerns or severe pain,

consider attending yoga classes led by experienced instructors or seeking guidance from a yoga therapist.

By integrating these yoga poses into your daily routine, you can effectively alleviate common pains, improve your flexibility, and enhance your overall sense of well-being. Yoga's gentle and holistic approach not only addresses physical discomfort but also promotes mental and emotional balance, leading to a healthier and more vibrant you. Remember to practice mindfully, respect your body's limitations, and enjoy the transformative benefits of yoga on your journey to pain-free living.

Breathing and meditation techniques for pain management

Pain is a universal human experience, but how we perceive and manage it can significantly impact our overall well-being. Breathing and meditation techniques provide powerful tools for managing pain, promoting relaxation, and enhancing our ability to cope with physical and emotional discomfort. By incorporating these practices into your daily routine, you can develop resilience, reduce stress, and find a sense of inner calm. Here's a comprehensive guide to breathing and meditation techniques for effective pain management:

1. Diaphragmatic Breathing (Deep Belly Breathing):

a. Technique:

Find a comfortable seated or lying position.

You should place one hand on either side of your abdomen and chest.

Allow your abdomen to balloon out as you take a deep, nasal inhalation.

Exhale slowly and completely through your mouth, feeling your abdomen deflate.

Make sure your chest is relatively motionless while concentrating on the rise and fall of your abdomen.

b. Benefits:

Diaphragmatic breathing promotes relaxation, reduces muscle tension, and calms the nervous system.

It enhances oxygenation, improving circulation and aiding in pain relief.

2. Mindful Breathing:

a. Technique:

Sit or lie down in a nice, quiet place.

Put your eyes closed and concentrate solely on your breathing.

Observe the natural inhalation and exhalation without trying to control it.

Refocus your attention on your breathing if your mind start to wander.

b. Benefits:

Mindful breathing enhances present-moment awareness, reducing anxiety and promoting a sense of calm.

It fosters acceptance of the present experience, including pain, without judgment or resistance.

3. Guided Imagery Meditation:

a. Technique:

Take a seat comfortably and shut your eyes.

Imagine a peaceful, serene place such as a beach, forest, or garden.

Engage all your senses: visualize the surroundings, feel the textures, hear the sounds, and smell the scents.

Immerse yourself in this mental sanctuary, allowing it to soothe your body and mind.

b. Benefits:

Guided imagery meditation distracts the mind from pain, reducing its perceived intensity.

It promotes relaxation, easing physical tension and discomfort.

4. Body Scan Meditation:

a. Technique:

Lie down in a quiet, comfortable space.

Close your eyes and bring your attention to different parts of your body, starting from your toes and moving upward.

Notice any sensations, tensions, or discomfort in each area without judgment.

Breathe into the areas of tension, allowing them to soften and relax.

b. Benefits:

Body scan meditation enhances body awareness, helping you identify and release areas of physical discomfort.

It promotes a sense of connection between your mind and body, fostering relaxation and pain relief.

5.   Loving-Kindness   Meditation   (Metta Meditation):

a. Technique:

Sit comfortably with your eyes closed.

Begin by sending loving and kind thoughts to yourself, such as "May I be happy. May I be healthy."

Gradually extend these thoughts to loved ones, acquaintances, and even people you have conflicts with.

Embrace all beings with feelings of love and compassion, wishing them happiness and freedom from suffering.

b. Benefits:

Loving-kindness meditation cultivates positive emotions, reducing negative emotions associated with pain.

It promotes empathy and compassion, fostering a sense of interconnectedness with others.

6. Breath Awareness with Mantra:
a. Technique:
Find a peaceful place to sit or to lie down.
Inhale deeply through your nose, silently repeating a calming word or phrase (mantra) in your mind.
Exhale slowly and completely, focusing on the rhythm of your breath and the mantra.
Let go of distracting thoughts, returning your focus to the mantra and your breath.
b. Benefits:
Breath awareness with mantra enhances concentration and mental clarity, calming the mind.
It promotes relaxation and reduces the perception of pain by redirecting the focus of the mind.

7. Walking Meditation:
a. Technique:
Find a quiet outdoor space or walk indoors in a peaceful environment.
Walk slowly and deliberately, focusing on each step and the sensation of your feet touching the ground.
Pay attention to your breath, syncing your inhalations and exhalations with your steps.
Engage your senses, noticing the sights, sounds, and smells around you as you walk.
b. Benefits:

Walking meditation provides gentle movement, promoting circulation and reducing stiffness.

It encourages mindfulness and relaxation, grounding you in the present moment and reducing pain-related stress.

Tips for Practicing Breathing and Meditation Techniques for Pain Management:

- **Consistency:** Practice regularly, ideally at the same time each day, to establish a routine and maximize the benefits.
- **Comfort:** Choose a comfortable posture and environment, ensuring you won't be disturbed during your practice.
- **Openness:** Approach these techniques with an open mind and a gentle attitude toward yourself, especially if you encounter challenges in your practice.
- **Professional Guidance:** Consider attending meditation or yoga classes led by experienced instructors to learn proper techniques and deepen your practice.
- **Patience:** Be patient with yourself. The benefits of breathing and meditation techniques often become more apparent with consistent practice over time.

By incorporating these breathing and meditation techniques into your daily life, you can effectively manage pain, reduce stress, and improve your overall quality of life. Remember that these practices are tools that empower you to navigate the challenges of pain with grace and resilience. As you cultivate a regular practice, you'll find inner calm and healing, leading to a more peaceful and harmonious relationship with your body and mind.

Partner stretches and massages for pain relief

Partner stretches and massages offer a unique and effective way to alleviate pain and promote relaxation. These practices not only provide physical relief but also strengthen emotional connections and trust between partners. By combining the healing power of touch with therapeutic stretches, you can create a harmonious environment that enhances well-being and reduces discomfort. Here's a detailed guide to partner stretches and massages for pain relief:

1. Partner Stretches:
a. Seated Forward Bend:
With your legs extended in front, sit facing your companion.
Extend your arms toward each other, holding hands or wrists.

Inhale and lengthen your spine, then exhale and gently fold forward, keeping your back straight.

Your partner can provide gentle resistance, enhancing the stretch. Hold for 20-30 seconds, breathing deeply.

b. Lower Back Twist:

On their backs, facing one another, the lovers both lie.

Put your feet level on the ground while bending your knees.

Cross your right leg over your left, then gently guide your partner's legs to the left side while keeping their shoulders on the ground.

Hold the stretch for 20-30 seconds, then switch sides.

c. Quad Stretch:

Partner A lies face down on the mat.

Partner B stands near Partner A's hips, holding their ankles.

Partner A bends their knees, and Partner B gently pulls their ankles toward their glutes, stretching the quadriceps.

Hold for 20-30 seconds, then release and switch roles.

d. Neck and Shoulder Stretch:

Sit or stand facing your partner.

Reach your right arm across your chest and place your hand on your partner's left shoulder.

Gently pull your partner's shoulder toward you, stretching the neck and upper back.

Hold for 20-30 seconds, then switch sides.

2. Partner Massages:

a. Neck and Shoulder Massage:

Sit behind your partner and gently squeeze their shoulders with your hands.

Use your thumbs to massage the sides of their neck, applying gentle pressure in circular motions.

Gradually increase pressure on tense areas and continue for 5-10 minutes.

b. Back Massage:

Partner A lies face down on the mat, and Partner B stands beside them.

Use your palms, knuckles, or elbows to apply long, gliding strokes along the muscles on either side of the spine.

Focus on areas of tension and use kneading motions to release knots gently.

Continue for 10-15 minutes, adjusting pressure based on your partner's preference.

c. Foot Massage:

Partner A sits comfortably with their feet elevated.

Partner B sits facing Partner A and uses oil or lotion to massage their feet and ankles.

Use your thumbs to apply circular motions on the soles, focusing on pressure points.

Gently stretch and rotate the ankles, providing relief to tired feet.

Continue for 10-15 minutes, ensuring both feet receive equal attention.

d. Hand and Wrist Massage:

Partner A sits comfortably, resting their hand on a cushion or pillow.

Partner B sits facing Partner A and uses oil or lotion to massage their hand and wrist.

Apply gentle pressure with your thumbs, focusing on the palm, fingers, and the area between the thumb and forefinger.

Perform circular motions and gently stretch the fingers and wrists.

Continue for 10-15 minutes, switching hands midway.

Tips for Partner Stretches and Massages:

- **Communication:** Maintain open communication with your partner. Ask for feedback regarding pressure, intensity, and areas of discomfort.
- **Warm-Up:** Warm-up your hands and apply gentle pressure initially to prepare the muscles for deeper stretches and massages.
- **Relaxation:** Create a relaxing environment with soft lighting, calming music, and comfortable cushions or mats.

- **Breathing:** Encourage your partner to breathe deeply and slowly during stretches and massages to enhance relaxation.
- **Trust:** Establish trust and respect boundaries. Always ask for consent before applying pressure, especially on sensitive areas.
- **Professional Guidance:** Consider attending workshops or classes on partner stretching and massage techniques to enhance your skills and knowledge.

Partner stretches and massages not only provide physical relief but also foster emotional intimacy and trust. By incorporating these practices into your routine, you can strengthen your bond with your partner while promoting relaxation and pain relief. Remember to approach these activities with patience, empathy, and mindfulness, allowing the healing power of touch to enhance your overall well-being and deepen your connection with your loved one.

Chapter 7

Chair Yoga for Mental and Emotional Well-being

Mindfulness and meditation exercises

In today's fast-paced world, the practice of mindfulness and meditation has gained significant recognition for its ability to reduce stress, enhance mental clarity, and promote overall well-being. These practices, rooted in ancient traditions, empower individuals to be fully present in the moment, fostering a deep sense of peace and inner strength. Here's a detailed guide to mindfulness and meditation exercises, offering a transformative journey toward greater self-awareness and emotional balance:

1. Mindful Breathing (Anapanasati):
a. Technique:
Look for a place that is calm and cosy to sit or to lie down.

Close your eyes and bring your focus to your breath.

Observe the natural rhythm of your breath, feeling the sensations as you inhale and exhale.

If your thoughts stray, gently and without passing judgement, bring them back to your breathing.

b. Benefits:

Mindful breathing calms the mind, reduces anxiety, and enhances focus and concentration.

It brings awareness to the present moment, promoting a sense of groundedness and tranquility.

2. Body Scan Meditation:

a. Technique:

Lie down in a comfortable position with your arms by your sides and eyes closed.

Bring your attention to your toes and gradually move upward, focusing on each part of your body.

In each location, pay attention to any sensations, tension, or relaxation. Breathe into areas of tension to release it.

Progressively scan your entire body, ending with the crown of your head.

b. Benefits:

Body scan meditation promotes body awareness, helping you identify and release areas of physical discomfort.

It encourages relaxation and a deep sense of connection between your mind and body.

3.   Loving-Kindness   Meditation   (Metta Bhavana):

a. Technique:

Lay down or take a seat comfortably.

Start by sending loving and kind thoughts to yourself, such as "May I be happy. May I be healthy."

Gradually extend these thoughts to loved ones, acquaintances, and even people you have conflicts with.

Embrace all beings with feelings of love and compassion, wishing them happiness and freedom from suffering.

b. Benefits:

Loving-kindness meditation cultivates positive emotions, reducing negative feelings and fostering self-compassion.

It enhances empathy and compassion toward others, strengthening social connections and promoting a sense of interconnectedness.

4. Walking Meditation (Kinhin):

a. Technique:

Find a quiet outdoor space or walk indoors in a peaceful environment.

Walk slowly and deliberately, focusing on each step and the sensation of your feet touching the ground.

Pay attention to your breath, syncing your inhalations and exhalations with your steps.

Engage your senses, noticing the sights, sounds, and smells around you as you walk.

b. Benefits:

Walking meditation provides gentle movement, promoting relaxation and reducing mental chatter.

It encourages mindfulness and presence, grounding you in the present moment and reducing stress.

5. Mindful Eating:

a. Technique:

Choose a piece of food (e.g., a raisin, nut, or fruit) and hold it in your hand.

Observe the food's texture, color, and aroma, engaging your senses fully.

Take a small bite and savor the taste and texture without rushing.

Notice the sensations as you chew and swallow, remaining present with each moment of the eating experience.

b. Benefits:

Mindful eating enhances your relationship with food, promoting healthier eating habits and preventing overeating.

It encourages gratitude for the nourishment your food provides, fostering a positive relationship with your body and diet.

6. Guided Meditation:

a. Technique:

Find a comfortable seated or lying position.

Use a meditation app to follow along or listen to a guided meditation recording.

Close your eyes and allow the guide's voice to lead you through a calming visualization or relaxation exercise.

Follow the instructions and immerse yourself fully in the experience.

b. Benefits:

Guided meditation offers structure and guidance, making it accessible for beginners and experienced practitioners alike.

It provides relaxation and stress relief, allowing you to surrender control and fully engage in the meditation process.

7. Mindfulness in Daily Activities:

a. Technique:

Choose a daily activity, such as washing dishes, taking a shower, or walking, to practice mindfulness.

Engage your senses fully in the activity, noticing the sensations, smells, and sounds associated with it.

Bring your full attention to each moment, resisting the urge to multitask or let your mind wander.

If your thoughts stray, gently bring your focus back to the activity without self-criticism.

b. Benefits:

Practicing mindfulness in daily activities cultivates presence and awareness in every aspect of your life. It reduces stress, enhances appreciation for simple moments, and promotes a sense of fulfillment in everyday tasks.

Tips for Practicing Mindfulness and Meditation:

- **Consistency:** Dedicate a specific time each day for your mindfulness and meditation practice to establish a routine.
- **Non-Judgment:** Approach your practice with an open, non-judgmental attitude. Be gentle with yourself and acknowledge any distractions without frustration.
- **Comfort:** Create a comfortable meditation space with cushions, blankets, or a supportive chair. Wear loose, comfortable clothing to allow free movement and relaxation.
- **Patience:** Progress in mindfulness takes time. Be patient with yourself, and embrace the journey without rushing.
- **Variety:** Explore different meditation techniques to find what resonates with you. There are various practices, such as body

scan, loving-kindness, and mantra meditation, catering to different preferences. By incorporating mindfulness and meditation exercises into your daily routine, you can cultivate a profound sense of presence, peace, and well-being. These practices provide invaluable tools to navigate life's challenges with grace and resilience. Remember that mindfulness is not about eliminating thoughts or emotions but about observing them without attachment. Through consistent practice and gentle dedication, you can embark on a transformative journey toward a more mindful, balanced, and harmonious life.

Yoga for stress reduction and relaxation

In the midst of our busy lives, stress often becomes a constant companion, affecting our physical and mental well-being. Yoga, an ancient practice that harmonizes the body, mind, and spirit, offers powerful tools for stress reduction and relaxation. Through a combination of gentle movements, breathing exercises, and mindfulness techniques, yoga provides a holistic approach to finding calm amidst chaos. Here's a detailed guide to using yoga as a means to reduce stress, promote relaxation, and foster overall well-being:

1. Mindful Breathing (Pranayama):

a. Deep Abdominal Breathing:

Select a comfortable sitting or lying position.

Place a hand on your chest and another on your stomach.

Inhale deeply through your nose, allowing your abdomen to rise and expand.

Feel your belly sag as you take a slow, mouth-exhale.

Focus on the gentle rise and fall of your breath, calming your mind and body.

b. Alternate Nostril Breathing (Nadi Shodhana):

Sit comfortably with your spine straight.

Use your right thumb to cover your right nostril and take a deep breath through your left nose.

Exhale via your right nostril while covering your left nose with your right ring finger.

Inhale deeply through your right nostril, then close it with your right thumb and exhale through your left nostril.

Continue this pattern, alternating nostrils. This exercise balances the energy channels in your body, promoting relaxation.

2. Yoga Poses (Asanas) for Stress Reduction:

a. Child's Pose (Balasana):

Kneel on the mat with your big toes touching and knees apart.

Lowering your forehead to the ground while leaning back on your heels and reaching your arms forward. Relax in this position, focusing on your breath and allowing your spine to lengthen.

b. Corpse Pose (Savasana):

Lie on your back with your legs extended and arms by your sides, palms facing up.

Close your eyes and take slow, deep breaths, releasing tension from each part of your body.

Visualize yourself in a peaceful place, such as a beach or a forest, allowing your body to fully relax.

c. Cat-Cow Pose (Marjaryasana-Bitilasana):

Start by putting your hands and legs together in a tabletop position.

Taking a breath in, elevate your head and tailbone while arching your back (Cow Pose).

Take a breath out, arch your back, and chin-tuck into the "Cat Pose."

Flow between these positions, syncing your breath with the movements to release tension in your spine.

d. Legs Up the Wall Pose (Viparita Karani):

Sit with your side against a wall, then gently swing your legs up the wall as you lie down.

Place your arms by your sides, palms facing up.

Close your eyes and focus on your breath, allowing your legs to relax against the wall. This pose promotes circulation and relaxation.

3. Mindfulness Meditation:

a. Technique:

Find a calm area and settle in with your back straight.

Focus on your breath by closing your eyes and paying close attention to each inhalation and exhalation.

If your thoughts stray, gently and without condemnation bring them back to your breathing.

Allow thoughts and emotions to come and go, practicing non-attachment and being fully present in the moment.

b. Benefits:

Mindfulness meditation cultivates awareness, reducing stress and anxiety by grounding you in the present moment.

It enhances your ability to respond to situations calmly, rather than reacting impulsively.

4. Guided Relaxation (Yoga Nidra):

a. Technique:

Lie down in a comfortable position with your legs extended and arms by your sides, palms facing up.

Close your eyes and follow the guidance of a yoga nidra recording or instructor.

The practice involves deep relaxation and visualization, systematically releasing tension from each part of your body.

b. Benefits:

Yoga nidra induces a state of profound relaxation, reducing stress and promoting deep rest.

It enhances sleep quality and supports overall well-being by allowing your body and mind to rejuvenate.

5. Gratitude Practice:

a. Technique:

Take a few deep, steady breaths to unwind while closing your eyes.

Reflect on three things you are grateful for, whether big or small.

Feel the gratitude in your heart and allow this positive emotion to fill your entire being.

b. Benefits:

Practicing gratitude shifts your focus from stressors to positive aspects of your life, fostering contentment and peace.

Promoting mental clarity and emotional resilience

In the face of life's challenges, nurturing mental clarity and emotional resilience is crucial. These qualities empower individuals to adapt, cope, and thrive in various situations, fostering a positive mindset and overall well-being. By cultivating mental clarity and emotional resilience, you can navigate stress, setbacks, and uncertainties with grace and inner strength. Here's a comprehensive guide to promoting mental clarity and emotional resilience:

1. Mindfulness Practices:
a. Mindful Breathing:
Practice deep breathing exercises, focusing on the inhalation and exhalation.

Be present in each breath, allowing your mind to settle and your body to relax.

Mindful breathing enhances awareness, promoting mental clarity and reducing stress.

b. Mindful Observation:
Observe your surroundings without judgment, noticing colors, shapes, and textures.

Engage your senses fully, appreciating the richness of your environment.

Mindful observation enhances focus and presence, fostering mental clarity.

c. Mindful Acceptance:
Practice acceptance of your thoughts and emotions without resistance.

Allow yourself to feel without judgment, acknowledging both positive and negative emotions.

Mindful acceptance reduces emotional reactivity, promoting resilience and inner peace.

2. Positive Self-Talk:
a. Challenge Negative Thoughts:
Identify your negative ideas and counter them with uplifting statements.
Replace self-criticism with self-compassion, acknowledging your worth and capabilities.
Positive self-talk fosters self-confidence and emotional resilience.
b. Practice Gratitude:
Regularly express gratitude for the people, experiences, and aspects of your life.
Keep a thankfulness diary and write down three things a day for which you are grateful.
Gratitude shifts focus to positive aspects of life, promoting mental clarity and emotional well-being.

3. Emotional Regulation:
a. Identify Triggers:
Recognize situations or people that trigger negative emotions.
Be mindful of your reactions and patterns of emotional responses.
Identifying triggers enables proactive coping strategies.
b. Breathwork and Relaxation Techniques:
Practice deep breathing, progressive muscle relaxation, or meditation during emotionally charged moments.

Use these techniques to calm the nervous system and regain emotional balance.

Breathwork and relaxation enhance emotional regulation and resilience.

4. Cultivating Emotional Intelligence:

a. Self-Awareness:

Reflect on your emotions, acknowledging and accepting them without judgment.

Understand the root causes of your feelings and their impact on your thoughts and behaviors.

Self-awareness enhances emotional intelligence and promotes resilience.

b. Empathy and Compassion:

Cultivate empathy by putting yourself in others' shoes and understanding their perspectives.

Practice compassion by extending kindness and understanding to yourself and others.

Empathy and compassion strengthen interpersonal relationships and emotional resilience.

5. Stress Management Techniques:

a. Regular Exercise:

Engage in physical activities like walking, yoga, or dancing.

Endorphins are released during exercise, which lowers stress and improves mental clarity.

Regular physical activity promotes emotional resilience.

b. Healthy Lifestyle Choices:

Prioritize sleep, nutrition, and hydration to support overall well-being.

Limit caffeine and alcohol intake, as they can affect mood and stress levels.

Healthy lifestyle choices provide a strong foundation for emotional resilience.

6. Effective Problem-Solving:

a. Identify Solutions:

Break down challenges into smaller, manageable parts.

Brainstorm potential solutions and consider their pros and cons.

Identifying solutions empowers you to take action, reducing feelings of helplessness.

b. Seek Support:

When faced with difficulties, seek the help of friends, family, or experts.

Sharing your concerns and seeking advice fosters a sense of connection and support.

Social support enhances emotional resilience by providing perspective and encouragement.

7. Practicing Mindful Communication:

a. Active Listening:

Practice active listening during conversations, fully focusing on the speaker without interrupting.

Validate the speaker's feelings and experiences, showing empathy and understanding.

Active listening promotes genuine connections and emotional resilience in relationships.

b. Expressing Emotions:

Communicate your feelings openly and assertively, using "I" statements to express your emotions without blame.

Be honest and clear about your needs, boundaries, and expectations.

Expressing emotions authentically fosters emotional resilience by promoting assertiveness and self-advocacy

Chapter 8

Chair Yoga for Specific Health Conditions

Chair yoga tailored for specific health issues

Chair yoga is a gentle and accessible form of yoga that can be modified to cater to various health conditions and physical limitations. Tailoring chair yoga practices to specific health issues, such as diabetes, heart conditions, osteoporosis, and more, allows individuals to enjoy the benefits of yoga while addressing their unique needs. Here's a comprehensive guide to chair yoga tailored for specific health issues, empowering individuals to enhance their well-being, regardless of their physical abilities:

1. Chair Yoga for Diabetes:
a. Gentle Warm-Up:
Seated neck rolls, shoulder stretches, and ankle circles promote circulation and flexibility.

Diabetic individuals should focus on warming up their joints and muscles to enhance blood flow.

b. Seated Forward Bend (Paschimottanasana):

Sit tall in a chair and place your feet firmly on the floor.

Inhale, lengthen your spine, and exhale, bending forward from your hips.

Hold the sides of the chair and relax into the stretch, promoting digestion and reducing stress.

c. Breathing Exercises:

Practice deep diaphragmatic breathing to enhance oxygenation and calm the nervous system.

Alternate nostril breathing (Nadi Shodhana) balances energy and promotes mental clarity.

2. Chair Yoga for Heart Conditions:

a. Chest Opener:

Sit comfortably, clasp your hands behind your back, and straighten your arms.

Inhale, lift your chest, and gently arch your back to open the heart center.

This pose improves lung capacity and circulation, supporting heart health.

b. Chair Pigeon Pose:

Place your feet flat on the ground while perched on the edge of a chair.

Cross your right ankle over your left knee, flexing your right foot.

Gently press down on your right knee to stretch your hips, promoting flexibility and reducing tension.

c. Guided Relaxation:

Use visualization techniques to imagine a peaceful place, promoting relaxation and stress reduction.

Relaxation poses like Savasana (Corpse Pose) can be adapted by sitting in the chair, focusing on deep relaxation and calming the mind.

3. Chair Yoga for Osteoporosis:

a. Seated Spinal Twist:

Put your feet firmly on the ground and sit tall in a chair.

Inhale, lengthen your spine, and exhale, twisting to the right and holding the back of the chair.

Twisting poses promote spinal flexibility and improve posture.

b. Leg Extensions:

Sit with your back straight and extend one leg forward, holding for a few breaths.

Lower the leg and switch sides. This strengthens leg muscles and promotes balance.

c. Wrist and Ankle Rotations:

Rotate your wrists and ankles gently in both directions to improve joint mobility.

These rotations maintain joint health, crucial for individuals with osteoporosis.

4. Chair Yoga for Arthritis:

a. Finger Stretch:

Extend your arms forward, spreading your fingers wide.

Gently stretch and flex your fingers, then make fists and release.

This helps maintain dexterity and relieves tension in the hands and wrists.

b. Chair Squats:

Stand behind a chair, holding onto it for support.

Lower into a squat position, keeping your knees aligned with your ankles.

Chair squats strengthen leg muscles, promoting stability and supporting joint health.

c. Breathing and Meditation:

Practice calming breathing exercises to reduce stress and anxiety.

Guided meditations focused on body awareness and relaxation can help manage pain and promote a sense of well-being.

5. Chair Yoga for Stress and Anxiety:

a. Deep Breathing Exercises:

Breathe in deeply through your nose and exhale slowly through your mouth to practise diaphragmatic breathing.

Progressive muscle relaxation involves tensing and releasing different muscle groups, promoting relaxation and reducing stress.

b. Chair Cat-Cow Stretch:

Place your hands on your knees as you sit in the chair.

Cow Pose: Breathe in, arch your back, and elevate your chest.

Take a breath out, arch your back, and chin-tuck into the "Cat Pose."

This gentle stretch promotes spinal flexibility and relaxation.

c. Meditation and Visualization:

Engage in guided meditation sessions focused on calming the mind and releasing tension.

Visualization exercises, such as imagining a peaceful beach or forest, can help reduce anxiety and promote mental clarity.

6. Chair Yoga for Multiple Sclerosis (MS):

a. Seated Mountain Pose:

Sit tall in the chair with your feet flat on the ground. Inhale, reach your arms overhead, and stretch upward.

This pose promotes balance and strengthens the core muscles.

b. Seated Leg Lifts:

Sit on the chair with your back straight and legs extended.

Lift one leg at a time, engaging your quadriceps, and hold for a few breaths.

Leg lifts improve leg strength and stability, supporting mobility.

c. Mindful Breathing and Body Scan:

Practice mindful breathing, focusing on the natural flow of your breath to enhance mental clarity and relaxation.

Body scan meditation helps you connect with your body, promoting awareness and acceptance of sensations and emotions related to MS.

Tips for Tailoring Chair Yoga:

- **Consultation:** Before starting any yoga practice, especially tailored for specific health issues, consult a healthcare professional or a qualified yoga instructor. They can provide personalized guidance based on your condition.
- **Awareness:** Listen to your body and honor its limitations. If a pose or movement causes pain or discomfort, modify or skip it.
- **Props:** Utilize props like cushions, belts, and yoga blocks to modify poses and enhance comfort and support.
- **Consistency:** Practice regularly, even if it's for a short duration. Consistency fosters

improvement in flexibility, strength, and overall well-being.

- **Mindfulness:** Approach each session with mindfulness, focusing on your breath, body sensations, and emotions. Mindful awareness enhances the benefits of yoga practice.

Chair yoga, tailored for specific health issues, empowers individuals to embrace the transformative benefits of yoga in a safe and accessible manner. By adapting poses and incorporating mindfulness techniques, individuals can enhance their physical and mental well-being, promoting a holistic sense of health and vitality.

Poses and practices to complement medical treatments

Integrating yoga poses and practices alongside conventional medical treatments can significantly enhance the healing process, promoting overall well-being and empowering individuals to actively participate in their recovery journey. Yoga offers a holistic approach, addressing not only the physical body but also the mind and spirit. Here's a comprehensive guide to yoga poses and practices that complement medical treatments, fostering healing and promoting a sense of balance and resilience:

1. Breathing Exercises (Pranayama):
a. Diaphragmatic Breathing:
Select a comfortable sitting or lying position.

By using your nose to breathe in, you can widen your diaphragm and fill your lungs with air.

Exhale slowly and completely through your mouth, allowing your abdomen to contract.

Diaphragmatic breathing calms the nervous system, reduces stress, and enhances oxygenation, supporting the body's healing process.

b. Alternate Nostril Breathing (Nadi Shodhana):
Sit comfortably with your spine straight.

Take a deep breath through your left nostril while covering your right nose with your right thumb.

Close your left nostril with your right ring finger, release your right nostril, and exhale completely.

This practice balances the energy channels in the body, promoting mental clarity and relaxation.

2. Gentle Yoga Poses:
a. Child's Pose (Balasana):
Kneel on the mat, sit back on your heels, and stretch your arms forward on the ground.

Rest your forehead on the mat and relax, focusing on deep, calming breaths.

Child's Pose gently stretches the spine, hips, and thighs, promoting relaxation and relieving lower back discomfort.

b. Cat-Cow Stretch (Marjaryasana-Bitilasana):

Start by getting down on your hands and knees, with your wrists under your shoulders and your knees under your hips.

Lift your head and tailbone in the "Cow Pose," inhaling as you arch your back.

Exhale, round your back, tuck your chin to your chest (Cat Pose).

Cat-Cow stretch promotes spinal flexibility, relieving tension in the back and neck.

c. Viparita Karani's Legs Up the Wall Pose:

Place your left side against the wall as you sit.

Lean back and swing your legs up against the wall so that your body forms an L.

Rest your arms by your sides with palms facing up, and close your eyes.

This gentle inversion promotes relaxation, improves circulation, and reduces swelling in the legs.

3. Meditation and Mindfulness:

a. Body Scan Meditation:

Lie down and close your eyes in a relaxed position.

Pay close attention to various body parts while observing sensations without passing judgement.

Breathe into areas of tension, allowing them to soften and relax.

Body scan meditation enhances body awareness, promoting relaxation and pain relief.

b. Loving-Kindness Meditation (Metta Bhavana):

Sit comfortably and close your eyes.

Start by sending loving and kind thoughts to yourself, then extend them to loved ones, acquaintances, and even challenging individuals.

Embrace all beings with feelings of love and compassion, wishing them happiness and freedom from suffering.

Loving-kindness meditation fosters positive emotions, reducing negative feelings and enhancing empathy.

4. Yoga Nidra (Yogic Sleep):

Lie down in a comfortable position with your arms by your sides and eyes closed.

Follow a guided Yoga Nidra meditation, focusing on relaxation and body awareness.

Yoga Nidra promotes deep relaxation, reducing stress and enhancing overall well-being.

5. Balancing Poses:

a. Tree Pose (Vrksasana):

Stand tall with your feet hip-width apart.

Shift your weight onto your left foot and lift your right foot, placing it on your inner left thigh or calf.

Alternatively, raise your arms aloft or bring your hands together in front of your chest.

Tree Pose improves balance, stability, and concentration.

b. Warrior Pose (Virabhadrasana):

Start in a standing position with your feet wide apart.

Turn your right foot out and bend your right knee, bringing your thigh parallel to the ground.

Stretch your arms parallel to the ground, palms facing down.

Warrior Pose strengthens the legs, promotes stability, and builds confidence.

Precautions and contraindications for various conditions

Yoga is a versatile and beneficial practice, but it's essential to approach it mindfully, especially if you have specific health conditions or injuries. Understanding precautions and contraindications related to various conditions is crucial to ensure a safe and effective yoga practice. Here's a comprehensive guide to help you navigate yoga with awareness, catering to your unique needs and circumstances:

1. Heart Conditions:

Precautions:

- Avoid intense or rapid movements that can spike your heart rate suddenly.
- Focus on gentle yoga styles, such as Hatha or Restorative yoga, emphasizing deep breathing and relaxation.
- Consult a healthcare provider before attempting inversions or intense backbends.

Contraindications:
- Avoid hot yoga or Bikram yoga, as excessive heat can strain the cardiovascular system.
- Skip poses that put significant pressure on the chest, like deep backbends or advanced twists.
- Pranayama techniques involving breath retention (Kumbhaka) should be avoided without professional guidance.

2. Pregnancy:
Precautions:
- Inform your yoga instructor about your pregnancy and attend prenatal yoga classes if possible.
- Avoid lying flat on your back after the first trimester; instead, use props to elevate your upper body for relaxation poses.
- Focus on gentle stretches, pelvic floor exercises, and breathing techniques to

promote relaxation and prepare for childbirth.

Contraindications:

- Avoid intense abdominal exercises, deep twists, and strong backbends, especially in the second and third trimesters.
- Skip inversions and poses that require balance, as the body's center of gravity shifts during pregnancy.
- Pranayama practices involving breath retention should be avoided.

3. Osteoporosis:

Precautions:

- Use props such as blocks and cushions to support your body and reduce strain on joints.
- Engage in gentle yoga styles focusing on slow, controlled movements to build strength and flexibility gradually.
- Practice balance poses near a wall or with a chair for support to prevent falls.

Contraindications:

- Avoid forward bends that put stress on the spine, especially from a standing position.
- Skip high-impact poses like jumping or poses that involve rapid and forceful movements.

- Poses requiring excessive flexion or extension of the spine, such as deep backbends, should be avoided.

4. Arthritis:
Precautions:
- Warm up thoroughly before practicing yoga, focusing on gentle joint movements to improve mobility.
- Use props and modify poses to accommodate your comfort level, ensuring proper alignment to prevent strain.
- Engage in gentle yoga styles like Yin yoga, focusing on longer holds and relaxation.

Contraindications:
- Avoid poses that cause pain or discomfort in your joints, especially weight-bearing poses like Plank or Downward Dog.
- Skip rapid and repetitive movements, as they can aggravate arthritis symptoms.
- High-impact activities or poses that put excessive stress on joints should be avoided.

5. Back Pain:
Precautions:
- Strengthen your core muscles to support the spine, focusing on poses that engage the abdominal muscles.

- Practice gentle backbends, such as Sphinx Pose, to improve flexibility in the spine.
- Use props like belts or yoga blocks to maintain proper alignment in seated or standing poses.

Contraindications:
- Avoid deep forward bends, especially with straight legs, as they can strain the lower back.
- Skip intense backbends or poses that cause discomfort in the spine, such as Wheel Pose or Camel Pose.
- Twisting poses that exacerbate back pain, especially without proper alignment, should be avoided.

6. Injuries (e.g., Sprains, Strains):
Precautions:
- Inform your yoga instructor about your injury, so they can guide you through modified poses.
- Practice gentle stretching and strengthening exercises to promote healing and prevent muscle imbalances.
- Listen to your body; if a pose causes pain or discomfort, back off and modify the position.

Contraindications:

- Avoid putting excessive pressure on the injured area; modify poses to avoid strain.
- High-impact activities and poses that exacerbate the injury, such as deep lunges or intense stretches, should be avoided.
- Consult a healthcare provider or physical therapist before resuming yoga practice after a significant injury.

7. Chronic Respiratory Conditions (e.g., Asthma, COPD):

Precautions:
- Focus on pranayama techniques that emphasize deep, controlled breathing, enhancing lung capacity.
- Practice gentle yoga styles, emphasizing relaxation and mindful breathing to reduce stress.
- Be mindful of your breathing during physical activities; if you experience shortness of breath, pause and rest.

Contraindications:
- Avoid practices in extreme temperatures or environments with poor air quality, as they can trigger respiratory symptoms.
- Skip intense breathing exercises like Kapalabhati, which may cause hyperventilation and exacerbate symptoms.

- Consult a healthcare provider before attempting practices involving breath retention or vigorous breathing.

General Precautions for All Practitioners:
- Stay hydrated before, during, and after your yoga practice to support the body's natural functions.
- Respect your body's limits and avoid pushing yourself into pain or discomfort; yoga is about self-care and self-awareness.
- Practice mindfulness and awareness, focusing on your breath and sensations in each pose.
- Listen to your body and rest when needed; fatigue or dizziness are signs to pause and recover.

Chapter 9

Chair Yoga for Daily Living

Incorporating chair yoga into daily routines

In today's fast-paced world, finding moments of tranquility and self-care is essential. Chair yoga, a gentle form of yoga practiced while sitting on a chair or using it for support, offers a perfect solution. It provides the benefits of traditional yoga, including improved flexibility, reduced stress, and enhanced mindfulness, without the need for a yoga mat or complicated poses. Here's a detailed guide on how to incorporate chair yoga into your daily routines, helping you infuse your day with calmness, balance, and rejuvenation:

1. Morning Mindfulness:
a. Seated Breath Awareness:
Start your day with a few minutes of seated breath awareness.
Sit comfortably in a chair with your feet flat on the ground and your hands resting on your lap.

Focus on breathing deeply through your nose and slowly out through your mouth while closing your eyes.

This practice calms the mind and sets a positive tone for the day.

b. Neck and Shoulder Stretches:

Gently tilt your head to the right, bringing your ear towards your shoulder, and hold for a few breaths.
Repeat on the left side.
Roll your shoulders forward and backward to release tension.
These stretches improve neck mobility and relieve shoulder stiffness.

2. Desk Breaks:

a. Seated Cat-Cow Stretch:
Sit with your feet flat on the ground and your hands on your knees.
Cow Pose: Breathe in, arch your back, and elevate your chest.
Take a breath out, arch your back, and chin-tuck into the "Cat Pose."
This seated version of Cat-Cow helps release tension in the spine and improves posture.

b. Chair Twists:
Sit tall in the chair with your feet flat on the ground.
Place your right hand on your left knee and your left hand on the backrest of the chair.

Inhale, lengthen your spine, and exhale, twisting gently to the left.

After a few breaths of holding, switch sides.

Chair twists improve spinal flexibility and promote digestion.

3. Lunchtime Relaxation:
a. Deep Breathing Exercise:

Take a break during your lunch hour for a deep breathing exercise.

Inhale deeply through your nose, expanding your lungs, and exhale slowly through your mouth.

Focus on your breath, allowing stress to melt away and promoting mental clarity.

b. Seated Forward Bend:

Place your feet firmly on the floor while sitting on the edge of your chair.

Inhale, lengthen your spine, and exhale, bending forward from your hips.

Reach your hands towards the floor or your shins, and hold the stretch for a few breaths.

Seated Forward Bend stretches your hamstrings and promotes relaxation.

4. Afternoon Energizer:
a. Chair Squats:

Stand up from your chair and position your feet hip-width apart.

Lower your body into a squat, as if you were about to sit back down.

Hold the position for a moment and then return to standing.

Chair squats strengthen your leg muscles and boost energy levels.

b. Seated Leg Lifts:

Sit at the front edge of your chair with your back straight.

Extend one leg forward, hold for a few breaths, and then lower it back down.

Switch sides and repeat.

Seated leg lifts improve leg strength and circulation.

5. Evening Relaxation:

a. Guided Meditation:

Find a quiet space, sit comfortably in your chair, and close your eyes.

Listen to a guided meditation session, focusing on relaxation and letting go of the day's stress.

Guided meditations promote mental calmness and prepare you for a restful night's sleep.

b. Seated Spinal Twist:

Sit tall in your chair with your feet flat on the ground.

Place your right hand on your left knee and your left hand on the backrest of the chair.

Inhale, lengthen your spine, and exhale, twisting gently to the left.

Hold the twist for a few breaths before reversing the position.

Seated spinal twists release tension in the back and promote relaxation.

6. Bedtime Wind-Down:

a. Relaxing Neck Stretches:

Sit or stand comfortably and tilt your head to the right, bringing your ear towards your shoulder.

Feel the stretch down your left side of your neck as you hold the position for a few breaths.

Repeat on the left side.

Neck stretches relieve tension built up during the day.

b. Deep Breathing and Progressive Relaxation:

Lie down in bed, close your eyes, and take a few deep breaths.

Focus on each part of your body, consciously relaxing and releasing any tension.

Start from your toes and work your way up to your head, promoting overall relaxation and preparing for sleep.

Tips for Successful Incorporation:

- **Consistency is Key:** Set aside specific times each day for your chair yoga practice, making it a consistent part of your routine.

- **Mindful Breathing:** Integrate deep breathing into your practice to enhance relaxation and focus.
- **Modify Poses:** Always modify poses according to your comfort level and physical condition, using props if needed.
- **Stay Hydrated:** Drink water throughout the day to stay hydrated, especially after your yoga sessions.
- **Respect Your Body:** Pay attention to the limitations of your body. Avoid pushing yourself into discomfort or pain.
- **Enjoy the Process:** Chair yoga is not just an exercise; it's an opportunity to connect with your body and mind. Enjoy the process and the sense of well-being it brings.

Incorporating chair yoga into your daily routines can transform your physical and mental well-being. By dedicating a few minutes at different points in your day, you infuse your routine with moments of calm and self-care. Whether it's a brief session at your desk or a guided meditation before bed, chair yoga offers a gentle path to relaxation and vitality, making each day a little more peaceful and balanced. Remember, your well-being is a journey, and chair yoga can be a delightful companion along the way.

Chair yoga for better sleep

Sleep is essential for overall well-being, yet many people struggle with getting sufficient rest. Chair yoga offers a gentle and effective solution to promote relaxation, reduce anxiety, and improve sleep quality. By incorporating chair yoga into your evening routine, you can create a tranquil bedtime ritual that signals your body and mind to unwind. Here's a comprehensive guide on how chair yoga can enhance your sleep, leading to nights of deep and rejuvenating rest:

1. Relaxation and Breathing Exercises:
a. Deep Breathing (Pranayama):
Sit comfortably in a chair with your feet flat on the ground and your hands resting on your lap.
Inhale deeply through your nose, expanding your lungs, and exhale slowly through your mouth.
Focus on your breath, allowing it to become slower and more rhythmic.
Deep breathing calms the nervous system, reducing stress and preparing your body for sleep.
b. Alternate Nostril Breathing (Nadi Shodhana):
Put your left hand on your left knee while maintaining a straight spine.
Use your right thumb to cover your right nostril and take a deep breath through your left nose.

Close your left nostril with your right ring finger, release your right nostril, and exhale slowly.
Repeat, alternating nostrils.
Nadi Shodhana balances the energy in your body, promoting relaxation and mental clarity.

2. Seated Stretches and Gentle Movements:

a. Neck Rolls:

Sit comfortably with your back straight and your hands resting on your thighs.
Slowly tilt your head to the right, then forward, to the left, and finally, backward, completing a full circle.
Perform a few rounds, reversing the direction.
Neck rolls release tension in the neck and shoulders, easing physical discomfort that might hinder sleep.

b. Shoulder Rolls:

Inhale, lift your shoulders towards your ears, and exhale, roll them back and down.
Repeat this movement, coordinating your breath with your shoulder rolls.
Shoulder rolls alleviate tightness in the upper back and shoulders, promoting relaxation.

3. Restorative Poses:

a. Supported Forward Bend:

Sit on the edge of a chair with your feet flat on the ground and your knees slightly apart.

Place a cushion or yoga block on your thighs and rest your forehead on it.

Hold the position, breathing deeply and letting go of tension.

Supported forward bend calms the mind, relieves stress, and soothes the nervous system.

b. Legs Up the Wall Pose (Viparita Karani):

Sit close to a wall with your side body touching it.

Swing your legs up the wall and descend your upper body to the floor at the same time.

Support your hips and lower back with a cushion or folded blanket.

Close your eyes and focus on your breath while holding the pose for a few minutes.

Legs up the wall pose promotes relaxation, relieves tired legs, and reduces anxiety.

4. Mindfulness Meditation:

a. Body Scan Meditation:

Lie down comfortably in your bed or on a yoga mat.

Close your eyes and bring your awareness to your toes.

Gradually move your attention up through each part of your body, noticing sensations without judgment.

Breathe into areas of tension, allowing them to soften and relax.

Body scan meditation promotes body awareness and relaxation, preparing your body for sleep.

b.   Loving-Kindness   Meditation   (Metta Bhavana):

Close your eyes as you sit or lie down in a comfortable position.

Begin by sending feelings of love and kindness to yourself, then extend those feelings to loved ones, acquaintances, and even challenging individuals.

Embrace all beings with feelings of love and compassion, wishing them happiness and freedom from suffering.

Loving-kindness meditation fosters positive emotions, reducing negative feelings and promoting relaxation.

5. Guided Relaxation Techniques:
a. Guided Visualization:

Close your eyes and imagine a peaceful and calming place, such as a beach or a forest.

Visualize the details – the colors, sounds, and scents of the environment.

Immerse yourself in this mental sanctuary, allowing your mind to wander and relax.

Guided visualization transports your mind to a serene place, helping you let go of daily concerns and prepare for sleep.

b. Yoga Nidra (Yogic Sleep):

Lie down comfortably with your arms by your sides and your eyes closed.

Follow a guided Yoga Nidra meditation, focusing on relaxation and body awareness.

Yoga Nidra promotes deep relaxation, reducing stress and enhancing overall well-being.

Tips for a Restful Sleep with Chair Yoga:

- **Consistent Practice:** Incorporate these chair yoga practices into your nightly routine, creating a consistent ritual before bedtime.

- **Create a Calm Environment:** Dim the lights, play soft, soothing music, and remove distractions to create a peaceful atmosphere conducive to relaxation.

- **Limit Screen Time:** Reduce exposure to electronic devices, such as smartphones or computers, at least an hour before bedtime to prevent overstimulation.

- **Comfortable Attire:** Wear loose, comfortable clothing to bed, ensuring you can move freely and feel relaxed.

- **Regular Sleep Schedule:** Aim for a regular sleep schedule, going to bed and waking up at the same time each day to regulate your body's internal clock.

- **Limit Caffeine and Stimulants:** Avoid consuming caffeine and stimulants in the evening, as they can interfere with your ability to fall asleep.

- **Stay Hydrated:** Drink water throughout the day, but limit intake closer to bedtime to prevent disruptions due to bathroom visits.
- **Consult a Professional:** If sleep difficulties persist, consider consulting a healthcare professional or a sleep specialist for further guidance.

By integrating chair yoga into your bedtime routine, you create a holistic approach to sleep, addressing both physical and mental aspects of relaxation. These gentle practices guide your body into a state of calm, easing stress and tension, and preparing you for a night of restorative sleep. Embrace these practices with patience and consistency, allowing the soothing benefits of chair yoga to enhance the quality of your sleep, and ultimately, your overall well-being. Remember, the path to better sleep begins with a single, tranquil breath.

Yoga practices for energy and vitality

In the hustle and bustle of modern life, finding sustainable energy and vitality is a universal pursuit. Yoga, an ancient practice that harmonizes the body, mind, and spirit, offers a holistic solution to boost your energy levels and enhance your overall vitality. By incorporating specific yoga practices into your routine, you can awaken your body, invigorate your spirit, and face each day with renewed vigor. Here's a detailed guide to yoga practices that promote energy and vitality, helping you tap into your inner reservoir of strength and enthusiasm:

1. Energizing Asanas (Poses):
a. Sun Salutations (Surya Namaskar):
Sun Salutations are a series of dynamic postures that warm up the body and increase circulation.
Practice several rounds in the morning to awaken your muscles, improve flexibility, and boost energy flow.
b. Warrior Poses (Virabhadrasana I, II, III):
These warrior poses build strength, stability, and confidence.
Engage your legs and core, allowing the empowering energy of the poses to infuse you with vitality.
c. Camel Pose (Ustrasana):
Camel Pose opens the chest and stimulates the respiratory and circulatory systems.
Practice this backbend to increase lung capacity, improve posture, and enhance overall energy levels.
d. Bridge Pose (Setu Bandhasana):
Bridge Pose strengthens the legs, buttocks, and lower back, promoting vitality in the lower body.
Hold the pose, breathing deeply, to awaken stagnant energy and increase vitality.

e. Chair Pose (Utkatasana):

Chair Pose strengthens the legs and core muscles, generating heat and energy in the body.

Engage your thighs and lift your chest, feeling the power and vitality coursing through your entire being.

2. Pranayama (Breath Control):
a. Kapalabhati (Skull Shining Breath):

Sit comfortably with a straight spine and exhale forcefully through your nose, followed by passive inhalation.

Kapalabhati increases oxygen supply, energizes the body, and clears the mind.

b. Nadi Shodhana (Alternate Nostril Breathing):

Sit in a comfortable position and use your right thumb to close your right nostril, inhaling deeply through your left nostril.

Close your left nostril with your right ring finger, release your right nostril, and exhale slowly.

Nadi Shodhana balances the energy channels, promoting mental clarity and vitality.

c. Ujjayi Pranayama (Victorious Breath):

Inhale deeply through your nose, slightly constricting the back of your throat to create a whispering sound.

Exhale slowly through your nose, maintaining the constriction to produce a gentle hissing sound.

Ujjayi Pranayama enhances concentration, calms the mind, and boosts energy levels.

3. Energizing Sequences:
a. Dynamic Flow Yoga:
Practice a flowing sequence, linking breath with movement, to build heat and energy in the body.
Incorporate sun salutations, warrior poses, and invigorating transitions to elevate your heart rate and boost vitality.
b. Power Yoga:

Power yoga combines strength-building poses with dynamic movements and continuous flow.
This vigorous practice challenges your body, increases stamina, and revitalizes your energy.

4. Meditation and Mindfulness:
a. Body Scan Meditation:
Lay down in a cosy position and start to become aware of various body areas.
Release tension and breathe into each area, allowing relaxation and vitality to flow through you.
b. Walking Meditation:
Take a mindful walk, focusing on your breath and the sensation of each step.
Connect with the energy of the earth beneath your feet, grounding yourself and absorbing revitalizing energy.

5. Energy-Balancing Mudras (Hand Gestures):
a. Prana Mudra:
Join the tips of your thumb, ring finger, and little finger, keeping the other two fingers extended.
Prana Mudra enhances the life force energy, revitalizing the body and increasing vitality.
b. Surabhi Mudra (Cow Gesture):
Curl your fingers into a fist, placing your thumbs inside your fingers.
Rest your hands on your thighs, feeling the grounding energy flow through your body.

6. Nutrition and Hydration:

a. Mindful Eating:
Consume whole, nutrient-dense foods, focusing on fruits, vegetables, whole grains, and lean proteins.
Stay mindful of portion sizes and eat slowly, savoring each bite to enhance digestion and energy absorption.
b. Hydration:
Stay hydrated throughout the day by consuming plenty of water to support your body's physiological processes.
Herbal teas and infused water with fruits and herbs add variety to your hydration routine.

7. Restorative Practices for Balance:

a. Pose with the Legs Up the Wall (Viparita Karani):

Lie down with your hips close to the wall and extend your legs upward, resting them against the wall.

Hold the pose, focusing on deep, calming breaths and allowing energy to flow back into your body.

b. Child's Pose (Balasana):

Kneel on the ground, sit back on your heels, and stretch your arms forward on the ground.

Rest your forehead on the mat and breathe deeply, surrendering tension and restoring your energy.

Tips for Integrating Yoga Practices for Energy and Vitality:

- **Consistency is Key:** Dedicate time for yoga regularly, whether it's a daily practice or several times a week, to experience the cumulative benefits.

- **Listen to Your Body:** Honor your body's limits and avoid pushing yourself into pain or strain. Yoga is about cultivating awareness and self-care.

- **Balanced Approach:** Combine energizing practices with restorative ones. Balance dynamic sequences with gentle stretches and meditation for a holistic approach to vitality.

- **Mindfulness:** Practice yoga with full presence, focusing on your breath, sensations, and the energy flowing within you. Mindfulness enhances the benefits of each pose and breath.

- **Professional Guidance:** If you're new to yoga or have specific health concerns, consider taking classes with experienced instructors who can guide you safely through the practices.

- **Quality Sleep:** Ensure you get sufficient rest. Quality sleep rejuvenates your body and mind, enhancing your overall vitality.

By embracing these yoga practices, you tap into your body's innate vitality, awakening your energy and cultivating a sense of well-being. With mindful movement, conscious breathing, and the power of intention, you can infuse your life with sustained vitality, enabling you to face each day with enthusiasm, clarity, and a revitalized spirit. Yoga becomes not just a physical practice, but a transformative journey that fuels your energy, empowering you to live life to the fullest.

Chapter 10

Building a Supportive Chair Yoga Community

Creating chair yoga groups and classes for seniors

Chair yoga offers a gentle and accessible way for seniors to enhance their physical and mental well-being. Creating chair yoga groups and classes for seniors not only promotes physical health but also provides a sense of community and support, fostering social connections and emotional well-being. Here's a comprehensive guide to help you create inclusive and enriching chair yoga sessions tailored specifically for seniors:

1. Understanding the Needs of Seniors:
a. Physical Considerations:
- Recognize common physical limitations, such as reduced flexibility, balance issues, and joint stiffness.

- Adapt yoga poses to accommodate these limitations, ensuring a safe and comfortable practice for seniors.

b. Mental and Emotional Well-Being:
- Be mindful of the emotional and mental challenges seniors may face, such as stress, anxiety, or depression.
- Incorporate relaxation techniques, breathing exercises, and mindfulness practices to address these concerns.

2. Obtaining Proper Certification and Training:

a. Yoga Certification:
- Obtain proper certification in chair yoga instruction, focusing on techniques and modifications suitable for seniors.
- Continuous education and workshops on senior-specific yoga practices are valuable for enhancing your expertise.

b. First Aid and CPR Certification:
- Consider obtaining first aid and CPR certification to ensure you can handle emergencies effectively during your classes.

3. Creating a Safe and Accessible Environment:

a. Choosing a Suitable Venue:
- Select a quiet, well-ventilated space with ample natural light, preferably free from distractions and noise.

- Ensure the venue is wheelchair accessible and has sturdy chairs without armrests for stability during yoga poses.

b. Using Props and Modifications:
- Provide props such as yoga blocks, straps, and cushions to support seniors in their practice.
- Offer modifications for poses, allowing participants to adapt movements based on their comfort and ability.

4. Designing Well-Structured Chair Yoga Classes:

a. Warm-up and Breathing Exercises:
- Begin with gentle warm-up exercises to prepare the body, incorporating joint movements and light stretches.
- Include breathing exercises (pranayama) to help participants relax and focus their minds.

b. Chair Yoga Poses:
- Choose a variety of seated and standing poses that improve flexibility, balance, and strength.
- Focus on poses that target common issues faced by seniors, such as back pain, arthritis, and joint stiffness.

c. Relaxation and Meditation:

- Include relaxation techniques, guided meditation, and mindfulness practices to promote mental calmness and emotional well-being.
- Guided imagery sessions can transport participants to peaceful and serene environments, enhancing their relaxation experience.

5. Fostering a Supportive Community:

a. Encouraging Social Interaction:

- Create opportunities for participants to interact and socialize before or after the class, fostering a sense of community.
- Organize occasional social events or outings to strengthen bonds among the members.

b. Listening and Responding:

- Actively listen to the participants' feedback and concerns, adjusting your classes accordingly to meet their needs.
- Provide a supportive and non-judgmental environment where seniors feel comfortable expressing themselves.

6. Promoting Safety and Well-Being:

a. Individual Assessments:

- Conduct individual assessments for new participants to understand their specific needs and limitations.

- Ensure participants are aware of their own limitations and encourage them to practice within their comfort zone.

b. Emergency Protocols:

- Have clear protocols in place for emergencies, including procedures for injuries, falls, or health-related issues.
- Keep emergency contact information for participants readily available and ensure your participants are aware of the procedures.

7. Marketing and Outreach:

a. Community Engagement:

- Engage with local senior centers, retirement communities, and community centers to promote your chair yoga classes.
- Offer free or discounted introductory sessions to attract participants and showcase the benefits of chair yoga.

b. Online Presence:

- Create a professional website and social media profiles to provide information about your classes, schedules, and testimonials.
- Use online platforms to share educational content, such as articles, videos, and infographics, related to chair yoga for seniors.

8. Feedback and Continuous Improvement:

a. Feedback Surveys:

- Regularly collect feedback from participants through surveys or open discussions.
- Use the feedback to make necessary adjustments to your classes, ensuring a positive and enriching experience for seniors.

b. Professional Development:

- Attend workshops, seminars, and conferences related to senior yoga and holistic well-being to enhance your teaching skills and knowledge.
- Stay updated with the latest trends and research in senior yoga to provide the best possible guidance to your participants.

By creating chair yoga groups and classes tailored for seniors, you're not only contributing to their physical health but also fostering a sense of belonging and connection within the community. Chair yoga becomes a conduit for enriching lives, promoting health, and enhancing the overall well-being of seniors, ensuring they lead vibrant and fulfilling lives. Remember, your passion, dedication, and compassion are key ingredients in creating a supportive and empowering chair yoga community for seniors.

Encouraging social interaction and support

Social interaction and support play a vital role in our overall well-being. Meaningful connections with others can boost our emotional, mental, and even physical health. Whether in local communities, workplaces, or online spaces, encouraging social interaction fosters a sense of belonging, reduces feelings of isolation, and provides a supportive network that can be invaluable in times of need. Here's a detailed guide on how to encourage social interaction and support, creating environments where individuals can thrive and communities can flourish:

1. Creating Inclusive Spaces:
a. Welcoming Atmosphere:
- Foster an environment of acceptance and inclusivity where everyone feels valued and respected.
- Encourage open-mindedness and celebrate diversity, embracing people from different backgrounds, cultures, and perspectives.

b. Accessible Venues:
- Ensure physical spaces are accessible to individuals with disabilities, accommodating various mobility needs.

- Provide clear signage and information to assist newcomers in navigating the environment comfortably.

2. Facilitating Meaningful Connections:
a. Icebreaker Activities:
- Incorporate icebreaker activities into events or gatherings to help people get to know each other.
- Icebreakers can include simple games, storytelling sessions, or collaborative projects that encourage interaction.

b. Group Activities and Workshops:
- Organize group activities, workshops, or classes that promote shared interests, such as art, gardening, cooking, or yoga.
- Collaborative projects foster a sense of camaraderie and provide opportunities for participants to engage with each other.

3. Encouraging Communication:
a. Active Listening:
- Cultivate active listening skills, encouraging individuals to express their thoughts, feelings, and concerns.
- Empathetic listening fosters trust and creates a safe space for people to open up.

b. Open Discussions and Forums:

- Host open discussions, forums, or town hall meetings where community members can voice their opinions, ideas, and suggestions.
- Transparent communication allows for collaborative problem-solving and strengthens community bonds.

4. Digital Communities and Social Media:
a. Online Support Groups:
- Establish online support groups or forums for specific interests, challenges, or goals.
- Online platforms provide a space for individuals to share experiences, seek advice, and offer support to others facing similar situations.

b. Engaging Social Media Content:
- Create engaging and positive content on social media platforms, encouraging discussions and interactions among followers.
- Thought-provoking questions, polls, and interactive posts stimulate conversations and strengthen online communities.

5. Volunteering and Community Service:
a. Community Service Projects:
- Organize volunteer initiatives that address local needs, such as clean-up drives, food

drives, or fundraising events for charitable causes.

- Participating in community service projects fosters a sense of pride and camaraderie among volunteers.

b. Skill and Knowledge Sharing:

- Encourage community members to share their skills, expertise, or hobbies with others through workshops or classes.
- Knowledge sharing not only benefits others but also strengthens the sense of community and mutual support.

6. Mentorship and Peer Support:

a. Mentorship Programs:

- Establish mentorship programs where experienced individuals guide and support newcomers or those facing specific challenges.
- Mentorship fosters a sense of belonging and provides valuable guidance and encouragement.

b. Peer Support Networks:

- Create peer support networks for individuals dealing with similar life events, such as illness, grief, or life transitions.
- Peer support provides a unique understanding and empathy, promoting healing and resilience.

7. Celebrating Achievements and Milestones:

a. Recognition and Appreciation:

- Acknowledge and celebrate individual and community achievements, both big and small.
- Recognition boosts self-esteem and motivates others, creating a positive atmosphere of appreciation.

b. Community Events and Festivals:

- Organize community events, festivals, or cultural celebrations that bring people together in a spirit of joy and unity.
- Shared celebrations strengthen community identity and create lasting memories.

8. Promoting Active Participation:

a. Leadership Opportunities:

- Provide opportunities for community members to take on leadership roles or contribute to decision-making processes.
- Empowering individuals enhances their sense of ownership and encourages active engagement.

b. Collaborative Projects:

- Facilitate collaborative projects where community members work together to address common challenges or pursue shared goals.

- Joint efforts foster a sense of pride and accomplishment, strengthening the community fabric.

9. Regular Feedback and Adaptation:
a. Feedback Mechanisms:
- Establish regular feedback mechanisms, such as surveys or suggestion boxes, to collect input from community members.
- Act on the feedback received, making necessary adjustments to enhance the community experience.

b. Adaptation and Flexibility:
- Remain adaptable and open to change, adjusting community initiatives based on evolving needs and preferences.
- Flexibility ensures that the community remains relevant and responsive to the dynamic nature of its members.

10. Promoting Empathy and Compassion:
a. Educational Workshops:
- Organize workshops or presentations on empathy, active listening, and compassionate communication.
- Providing tools for understanding and empathy strengthens interpersonal relationships within the community.

b. Encouraging Acts of Kindness:

- Encourage random acts of kindness within the community, promoting a culture of compassion and support.
- Small gestures can have a significant impact, creating a ripple effect of kindness and empathy.

By encouraging social interaction and support within communities, we nurture environments where individuals feel valued, connected, and empowered. These connections not only enhance personal well-being but also contribute to the overall strength and resilience of the community. The bonds formed through social interaction and support serve as a foundation for a compassionate, inclusive, and thriving society, where individuals are empowered to navigate life's challenges with the strength of community behind them. Remember, every smile, every shared story, and every act of kindness strengthens the fabric of community, weaving a tapestry of support and belonging for all.

Conclusion

Recap of key lessons and practices

Embarking on the path of personal growth and well-being involves embracing key lessons and practices that enrich our lives, foster resilience, and deepen our sense of fulfillment. As we reflect on our journey, let's recap the essential lessons and practices that form the foundation of a meaningful and purposeful life:

1. Self-Compassion and Acceptance:
Lesson: Embrace yourself with kindness, acknowledging your strengths and embracing your imperfections.
Practice: Cultivate self-compassion through mindfulness, meditation, and positive self-talk. Treat yourself with the same kindness you would offer a dear friend.

2. Mindfulness and Present Moment Awareness:
Lesson: The present moment is where life unfolds. Embrace it fully, free from judgment and distraction.

Practice: Practice mindfulness meditation, grounding exercises, or simply paying full attention to everyday tasks. Presence cultivates clarity, reduces stress, and enhances overall well-being.

3. Gratitude and Positivity:

Lesson: Gratitude transforms ordinary moments into extraordinary blessings, fostering a positive outlook on life.

Practice: Keep a gratitude journal, regularly noting down things you are thankful for. Express gratitude to others, fostering meaningful connections and spreading positivity.

4. Healthy Lifestyle Choices:

Lesson: Nourish your body, mind, and soul with wholesome nutrition, regular exercise, and sufficient rest.

Practice: Prioritize balanced meals, engage in physical activities you enjoy, practice relaxation techniques, and ensure quality sleep. A healthy lifestyle fuels vitality and supports overall well-being.

5. Emotional Intelligence and Relationships:

Lesson: Understanding and managing your emotions empowers meaningful, empathetic connections with others.

Practice: Practice active listening, empathetic communication, and emotional regulation. Cultivate genuine relationships, where understanding and support flow freely, nurturing your emotional well-being.

6. Resilience and Adaptability:

Lesson: Life's challenges are opportunities for growth. We can face misfortune with elegance and courage when we are resilient.

Practice: Develop a growth mindset, embracing challenges as learning experiences. Practice resilience through meditation, affirmations, and seeking support from loved ones.

7. Purpose and Meaning:

Lesson: Discovering your purpose gives life profound meaning and direction, fueling your passion and creativity.

Practice: Reflect on your passions, strengths, and values. Set meaningful goals aligned with your purpose, and engage in activities that align with your passions, contributing positively to your community and the world.

8. Compassion and Acts of Kindness:

Lesson: Compassion is a powerful force that connects us, fostering understanding, kindness, and unity.

Practice: Perform acts of kindness regularly, whether small or significant. Volunteer, help a neighbor, or simply offer a listening ear. Compassion ripples outward, creating a positive impact on the world.

9. Mind-Body Connection and Holistic Wellness:

Lesson: Our mental and emotional well-being profoundly influence our physical health. Integrating the mind, body, and spirit is holistic wellness.

Practice: Engage in practices that promote mind-body harmony, such as yoga, meditation, tai chi, or deep breathing exercises. Nurture your spiritual well-being through mindfulness, prayer, or connecting with nature.

10. Continuous Learning and Growth:

Lesson: Embrace a lifelong journey of learning and self-discovery, expanding your horizons and evolving as an individual.

Practice: Read books, take courses, learn new skills, and engage in activities that challenge your mind. Seek inspiration from diverse sources, fostering intellectual curiosity and personal growth.

11. Gracious Self-Reflection and Self-Care:

Lesson: Regular self-reflection enhances self-awareness, guiding your path toward fulfillment and authenticity.

Practice: Journal your thoughts and feelings, reflecting on your experiences and insights. Prioritize self-care activities that bring you joy and relaxation, ensuring your well-being remains a top priority.

12. Connection with Nature:

Lesson: Nature is a source of profound healing and inspiration, grounding us in the beauty and tranquility of the natural world.

Practice: Spend time outdoors, whether in a park, garden, or natural reserve. Engage in nature walks, meditate under trees, and connect with the elements. Nature renews the spirit and fosters a sense of awe and wonder.

As we incorporate these key lessons and practices into our lives, we embark on a transformative journey toward holistic well-being. Each step we take, each moment of mindfulness, and each act of kindness contributes to a life rich in meaning and purpose. Remember, this journey is uniquely yours, and every experience, whether joyful or challenging, holds valuable lessons that shape your growth. Embrace each day with gratitude, curiosity, and an open heart, for within these moments lie the seeds of your personal evolution and enduring happiness.

Encouragement for ongoing chair yoga practice

Embarking on a chair yoga practice is a transformative journey toward enhanced well-being, flexibility, and inner peace. As you step onto this path, it's essential to nurture your commitment and enthusiasm for regular practice. Here's a comprehensive guide offering encouragement and valuable tips to support your ongoing chair yoga journey:

1. Celebrate Progress, Big and Small:

Encouragement: Acknowledge and celebrate your progress, no matter how small it may seem. Every chair yoga session, every stretch, and every deep breath is a step toward improved health and vitality.

Tip: Keep a journal to record your achievements and milestones. Reflect on how your body feels after each session, noticing any improvements in flexibility, balance, or overall well-being.

2. Embrace Consistency:

Encouragement: Consistency is the key to reaping the full benefits of chair yoga. Regular practice creates a positive routine, promoting physical and mental well-being.

Tip: Set a specific time each day or several times a week dedicated to chair yoga. Make it a non-negotiable part of your schedule, just like any other important activity.

3. Listen to Your Body:

Encouragement: Your body is your best guide. Listen to its signals and honor its limitations. Chair yoga is about gentle progression and self-compassion.

Tip: Pay attention to how your body feels during and after each pose. If you experience discomfort or pain, modify the pose or skip it entirely. Always prioritize your comfort and well-being.

4. Explore Variations and New Poses:

Encouragement: Chair yoga offers a vast array of poses and modifications. Explore different variations to keep your practice exciting and engaging.

Tip: Experiment with new poses and modifications you discover online, in books, or during classes. Embrace the opportunity to expand your practice and challenge yourself gently.

5. Incorporate Mindfulness and Breathwork:
Encouragement: The union of breath and movement is the essence of yoga. Practice mindfulness and deep breathing to enhance your chair yoga experience.
Tip: Focus on your breath during each pose, inhaling and exhaling mindfully. Notice the sensation of the breath filling your lungs and the calming effect it has on your mind. This mindful approach deepens your practice.

6. Join Chair Yoga Communities:
Encouragement: Connecting with like-minded individuals can boost your motivation and enthusiasm for chair yoga. Online forums, local classes, or social media groups provide supportive communities.
Tip: Join online chair yoga forums or social media groups to share your experiences, ask questions, and learn from others. Engaging with a community fosters a sense of belonging and encouragement.

7. Reward Yourself:

Encouragement: Acknowledge your commitment to chair yoga by rewarding yourself for reaching milestones or sticking to your practice routine.
Tip: Set achievable goals, such as practicing chair yoga three times a week for a month. When you

reach your goal, treat yourself to something special—a favorite healthy snack, a relaxing bath, or a new yoga accessory.

8. Stay Curious and Open-Minded:
Encouragement: Approach your chair yoga practice with curiosity and an open mind. Each session is an opportunity to learn more about your body and its capabilities.
Tip: Attend different chair yoga classes, watch instructional videos, or read books on the topic. Embrace the wealth of knowledge available, allowing your practice to evolve and grow.

9. Be Patient and Kind to Yourself:
Encouragement: Progress in chair yoga, like any form of yoga, takes time and patience. Be kind to yourself, embracing the journey with self-compassion.
Tip: Practice patience and self-acceptance. Understand that progress might be slow, but each effort is a step in the right direction. Treat yourself with the same kindness you would offer a dear friend.

10. Celebrate Your Commitment:
Encouragement: Your commitment to chair yoga reflects your dedication to your well-being.

Celebrate this commitment as a powerful act of self-love and self-care.

Tip: Reflect on how chair yoga positively influences your life. Notice the improvements in your physical health, mental clarity, or emotional balance. Celebrate these changes, affirming your dedication to your own well-being.

By embracing these encouragements and tips, your chair yoga practice becomes a nurturing and empowering journey. Remember, your dedication to your well-being is a precious gift to yourself. With each stretch, each breath, and each moment of mindfulness, you're investing in your health and vitality, fostering a sense of inner harmony and balance. May your chair yoga practice continue to bring you joy, strength, and a profound connection with your own body and spirit. Namaste.